IMPO...
Sexually ...

Chlamydia—The ... in the U.S., with three to ten million cases a year. Known as the "silent epidemic"—the disease produces no symptoms for weeks to months, and sometimes not for years. Both men and women can be infected. Routine testing is advised. It can be effectively treated and cured with antibiotics.

Syphilis—A dramatic increase in reported cases in 1987. It is highly contagious, but easily cured with penicillin in the *early* stages.

Gonorrhea—Approximately two million cases reported each year in the U.S., but the real incidence of infection may actually be twice as high. It can remain "silent" in women, producing no symptoms. Cured quickly, if treated early.

Genital Warts—The most common *viral* STD, with approximately three million new cases reported every year. They are not only contagious but can be a serious health threat to both men and women and require medical treatment.

PID (Pelvic Inflammatory Disease)—An infection of the reproductive tract in women. It is the end result of other STDs, such as gonorrhea and chlamydia, if these diseases go untreated. PID can cause inflammation of all the upper reproductive organs, and the resulting scarring can cause tubal pregnancies, miscarriages, and infertility.

GET THE FACTS AND PROTECT
YOURSELF WITH . . .
A WOMAN'S GUIDE TO SEXUAL HEALTH

A WOMAN'S ·G·U·I·D·E· TO SEXUAL HEALTH

Sue DeCotiis, M.D.

POCKET BOOKS

New York   London   Toronto   Sydney   Tokyo

This book is intended to supplement, not replace, the advice of your doctor. If you know or suspect that you have a health problem, you should consult a trained health professional.

An *Original* Publication of POCKET BOOKS

 POCKET BOOKS, a division of Simon & Schuster Inc.
1230 Avenue of the Americas, New York, NY 10020

Copyright © 1989 by Dr. Sue G. DeCotiis

ISBN: 0-671-66011-X

First Pocket Books printing October 1989

10 9 8 7 6 5 4 3 2 1

POCKET and colophon are trademarks of Simon & Schuster Inc.

Printed in the U.S.A.

Contents

CONTENTS

Author's Preface

Sexually transmitted diseases (STDs) cause special problems for women. They are usually difficult to recognize and, if untreated, can lead to infertility or serious illness. The media tend to address STDs from a male point of view, failing to explain many of the special issues of diagnosis and treatment that are crucial to women. For these reasons, knowing more about how your body works and what to look for is important. *A Woman's Guide to Sexual Health* provides the detailed information you won't find in a magazine or newspaper article, not only on the diseases themselves, but also on the particular issues and choices we face every day about things like safe sex, birth control, pregnancy, and good sexual health.

Every year STDs infect large numbers of women, but they don't have to, since most STDs are avoidable. Though many STDs aren't life-threatening, the tragedy is that some women will become infertile from pelvic disease that can follow the original infection. Others may pass on a disease to their unborn or newly born children, and this can often be serious. And some STDs are very harmful indeed; the AIDS virus is fatal in a majority of those who have it, and some kinds of genital warts are believed to cause cervical cancer. Finally, getting any disease is upsetting, but getting a sexually transmitted disease can be doubly so, with often unfortunate consequences for a relationship, either new or established.

I wrote this book so that women might have a reference that would explain the most common kinds of sexual disease clearly and completely. *A Woman's Guide to Sexual Health* offers detailed discussions of more than thirty common STDs, together with information on their symptoms, diagnosis, treatment, transmission, and prevention.

There is a complete chapter on AIDS, addressing women's concerns in the light of what we know today. The latest information on risk groups, how the virus can be transmitted, and advice for assessing your risk is included. "Safe Sex," Chapter 9, teaches you not only how to have safer sex but also what is safe and why so that you can make informed choices to protect your sexual health. In "Birth Control," the last chapter, you will learn how the kind of birth control you use can play a big role not only in preventing pregnancy, but in protecting you against STDs, too.

The book's organization generally follows a woman's anatomy from the outside in. Diseases causing lesions on the outer genitals are covered first; then diseases of the lower and upper pelvic organs; then viral diseases. The final chapters of the book cover

AIDS and other viral diseases, safe sex, and birth control.

Most of the book is written in a question-and-answer format. If you are looking up a specific disease, however, I would suggest you also read the anatomy section relevant to it. For example, reading the anatomy section at the start of Chapter 1 will help you become familiar with how things work and the terms used in the pages that follow. Nearly every disease is also followed by two important sections: "Special Considerations" and "If You Have . . ." The first informs you about the disease as it relates to pregnancy, cancer, and other things you need to know. The second tells you what you should do and should not do so you can be as comfortable as possible before and during treatment but not pass the disease on to someone else before you're cured.

The glossary will help you find quick definitions for the many new medical terms you will be learning throughout the book. It is organized alphabetically and includes all of the words you will need to know as you read along.

Finally, I cannot overemphasize the importance of regular checkups and annual Pap tests for your good sexual health. Armed with the background this book provides, you will be able to work with your doctor to safeguard your health and the health of those you love.

FIGURE 1:
The Vulva

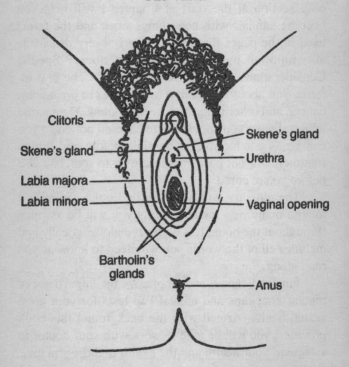

Clitoris

Skene's gland

Skene's gland

Urethra

Labia majora

Labia minora

Vaginal opening

Bartholin's
glands

Anus

PART
I
Genital Lesions

S ome of the most common sexually transmitted diseases are those that appear on the external sex organs or genitalia, which in women are called the vulva. These include diseases most people have heard of like **herpes simplex,** and others like **genital warts,** the most common STD diagnosed today though many people haven't heard of it.

Genital Lesions: An Overview

Often, the first sign that you have an STD is a bump, blister, ulcer, or sore—collectively known as "lesions." These lesions may appear suddenly or gradually on your genitals, and you may notice them for the first time while bathing, using the bathroom, or during intimacy.

Learning about the diseases that cause genital lesions helps you to recognize them in a potential partner and thus avoid contracting them. You will know what to look for if you suspect you may have one. You won't panic when you discover a sore (having read about traumatic lesions and remembering too-tight jeans that chafed), and you will know how serious certain lesions can be, what the treatment is, and how to get it. You can also avoid giving them to someone else while waiting for treatment. Most importantly, knowing what causes such lesions and how to prevent them reduces your chances of ever getting one in the first place.

Genital lesions are caused by many common STDs. They may appear suddenly or develop slowly over a period of time. They may be painful, and quickly discovered, or painless, in which case you might only notice one by accident, while bathing or dressing. Since a woman's genitals are "hidden"—certainly less obvious than the completely external male penis—you should examine your genitals with a mirror regularly, just as you might do a monthly breast self-exam.

Genital lesions can be identified by their appearance. An **ulcer**—what we call a "sore"—is a loss of the top layers of skin, which creates a depression on the surface, often exposing the raw and pinkish layers of tissue beneath. Depending on the disease causing them, ulcers can vary greatly in size, shape, depth, and the pain they cause you. Ulcers are most often involved in **herpes, syphilis,** and **traumatic lesions** and rarer diseases like **chancroid.**

Other genital lesions, unlike ulcers, can be *raised*. They sit on top of the skin and may look like bumps, pimples, or rough patches. STDs that cause raised lesions include genital warts, Bartholin's duct infection, molluscum contagiosum, scabies, and pubic lice.

CHAPTER ONE

Common Genital Lesions

The Anatomy of the External Genitals

To begin to learn the basics of the genital anatomy, you might want to do a self-exam. Take a hand mirror and hold it in front of your genitals with your pelvis tilted slightly forward so you can see the image.

From the outside in, the vulva consists of the labia majora, the labia minora, the clitoris, and the urethral and vaginal openings.

The labia majora (Latin for "major lips") are the two outermost large folds or lips of skin-colored fatty tissue; they protect and partially cover the vaginal and urethral openings. The labia majora are covered, on the outside, with coarse and thick pubic hair, which absorbs moisture. The smooth, hairless inner surface of the labia majora is lined with thin, delicate pink tissue—mucous membrane tissue like that also found inside your mouth and nose and on your nipples.

The labia minora ("small lips") are the two smaller folds of mucous membrane tissue found inside the labia majora. The labia minora guard the vaginal and urethral openings even more closely than the labia majora. Toward the top, the labia minora merge at the clitoris, a fleshy knob of sensitive tissue with many nerve endings, which, like the male penis, can become erect when filled with blood during sexual excitement.

Beneath the clitoris, between the two folds of the labia minora, is the urethral opening, where the urethra—the thin tube that carries urine from the bladder—empties. Around the urethral opening are two tiny glands called Skene's glands, which lubricate the urethral opening. Skene's glands only become noticeable when infected.

Under the urethral opening is the larger vaginal opening, which is ringed with strong, elastic muscles. These elastic muscles allow the vagina to expand greatly to accommodate a penis during intercourse or to allow the passage of a baby during birth. Surrounding the vaginal opening are the pea-sized Bartholin's glands, which produce small amounts of lubricating fluid to prepare the vagina for sexual intercourse. These glands, like the Skene's glands, are usually not noticeable unless they become infected and swell up.

Except for the outer surface of the labia majora, the entire vulva is lined by mucous membrane, delicate tissue that receives a large blood supply, is moist, and is usually not exposed to light—all characteristics that make the vulva extremely vulnerable to infection by STDs.

TRAUMATIC LESIONS

The most common cause of genital lesions is not an STD at all, but rather the minor injuries or irritations of everyday life. This type of lesion is called a **traumatic lesion** and could be a slight scratch or scrape on the surface of the skin like when you scrape a knee. There may be redness, itchiness, or a chafed spot on the surface of the skin. Vigorous or prolonged intercourse or masturbation (especially when there is little or no lubrication), overuse of sex tools like vibrators, and tight pantyhose or underwear are all causes of traumatic lesions. Sometimes the irritation will be enough to cause a sore to form, especially if the irritation continues and you scratch it.

Though this minor irritation of the skin of the vulva may be uncomfortable, don't worry, especially if any of the causes listed here sound familiar to you. In the meantime, wash your genitals with mild soap and don't scratch if it itches. These harmless lesions usually heal themselves in two or three days without medication.

If, after three days, you're still uncomfortable and the lesion has not healed, or if you are unsure what caused the irritation, you should call your doctor. Even though it may turn out to be harmless, don't wait to call—make sure you're okay.

If the lesion doesn't heal and you do see a doctor, she may prescribe an antibiotic ointment to be applied to the lesion, which will usually then heal in a week. If the lesion is still there, your doctor may want to do further tests to determine if it is a symptom of any of the STDs covered in the rest of this chapter.

If a traumatic lesion is scratched or is not kept clean, it can become infected by the bacteria normally present in the genital area. If this happens, the lymph glands or nodes in the groin can become swollen and tender. The swollen glands together with the sore may look like a more serious genital lesion. (The lymph nodes are small, round masses of glandular tissue on either side of the inner thighs where they meet to form a V. The lymph nodes drain impurities from body tissue during infection.) When you do go to the doctor for a sore that hasn't healed, she will first want to make sure the sore is not a symptom of more serious diseases like syphilis and herpes. If your doctor feels the lesion is infected, she may prescribe antibiotics like Keflex or tetracycline pills for a week.

If you have a traumatic lesion:

- don't use greasy skin emollients or creams; they can help cause infection.
- don't use steroid or cortisone creams without your doctor's approval. These creams slow healing and can encourage further infection. It is fine to use steroid or cortisone cream in combination with antibacterial medication with your doctor's supervision.
- see your doctor if the sore doesn't heal after three days.
- avoid the source of irritation—tight clothes, vibrators, or lack of lubrication during sex.

GENITAL HERPES

What is genital herpes?

Genital herpes is a highly contagious, incurable STD caused by the virus Herpes simplex virus 2, or HSV2. It is currently the third most common STD in heterosexuals and has infected more than twenty million Americans, with about 200,000 new cases reported every year. A person infected with genital herpes develops painful genital ulcers, or sores, which heal but reappear periodically over many years following the initial outbreak. It can be treated but not cured and lives on in the body. Genital herpes is long-term and is contagious and painful during each recurrence; it thus restricts your sex life to periods when it is noncontagious. Herpes can cause complications in pregnancy (miscarriage and premature birth) and serious illness (pneumonia) in babies born to infected mothers. In addition, research has shown that if you have herpes, you may be more likely to develop cancer of the cervix or, less commonly, cancer of the vulva.

How long does it take for the first symptoms of genital herpes to appear?

After exposure to the herpes virus it can take anywhere from one week to as long as a month before you notice anything. Usually, however, the first symptoms begin about one week after exposure. This first appearance of symptoms is called the initial attack.

How do I know if I have herpes? What are the symptoms?

When a woman has an initial attack of herpes, she usually has very painful symptoms that can last up to three weeks. Often, the first symptom is a numbness, tingling, or burning/stinging sensation in your vulva as the virus irritates the nerves in the lower genital tract. You may feel a burning sensation when you urinate and/or pain during intercourse. At the same time or within a few days, from one to twenty soft red bumps varying in size from barely visible to a half inch in diameter may appear on your vulva. These bumps will appear on the outer and inner lips, urethral opening, clitoris, and around the anus or on the buttocks. The bumps pop up, becoming raised blisters filled with a small amount of fluid. Herpes blisters only occur during the first attack. At this point, they look like white, pimply patches and cause sharp, shooting, or burning pain. Since the fluid is laden with the herpes virus, these white patches are highly contagious and can give your sex partner herpes very easily.

Two or three days after the blisters form they break down and make an ulcer in the same place and of the same size as the blister. But while the blister was raised, the ulcer is sunken and wet and has smooth edges. The herpes ulcer looks like a worn-away spot exposing the pink, raw tissue underneath. The ulcers are as painful and contagious as the blisters and usually heal within seven to ten days, leaving little or no scarring.

Blisters and ulcers can also appear in the vagina and cervix, where there are few nerve endings and no pain is felt. If there are no other blisters or ulcers on the vulva, the disease may go untreated, since you can't see anything and nothing hurts.

From the first appearance of the red bumps to the final healing of the white patches and ulcers, the first attack usually lasts from twelve to fourteen days, though in some people the ulcers can take as long as three weeks to heal. It is very painful, and even the touch of something as light as a bedsheet can be torture. Other, less common symptoms that sometimes appear are fever, tiredness, headache, and enlargement of the lymph nodes in the groin. These symptoms tend to be more severe (and more painful) in women than in men.

Are the symptoms different for a man? How can I tell if my partner has it?

In men, the blisters and ulcers appear just as they do in women, except that they can appear anywhere on the penis and/or on the anus, buttocks, or scrotum. The ulcer that follows the blister tends to be drier in men, and often less painful, too, although just as contagious. Men can also experience the secondary symptoms—fever, fatigue, and headache.

One way to tell if a man has herpes is to ask him. Unfortunately, his answer may not be truthful for two reasons: He may not want to tell you, or he may be infected and not know it himself. You can check this out for yourself: Look closely before any skin-to-skin contact, even embracing, for the blisters, red spots, and sores described above. If you're still not sure, ask him to have a checkup before you have intimate contact, and tell him you will, too.

How do you get herpes?

Most people get herpes from sexual contact with someone already infected with the disease. Often, but not always, the infected person will have ulcers on his or her genitals, sores not always visible to either partner that contain highly contagious particles of the herpes virus. Herpes is highly contagious in all its states from the appearance of the initial red spots (from one week to one month after exposure) until the white bumps or patches that form the ulcer heal completely. Herpes is contagious during the first attack and during every subsequent recurrent attack. Most often, herpes heals completely, leaving no scar.

Do you always have symptoms with a herpes infection?

Some people with herpes never develop sores or blisters but can give it to you through contact with small flakes of their genital skin, semen, or vaginal fluids or secretions. This means that someone can pass on the disease without ever knowing they have it. People who can do this are called "asymptomatic shedders." This shedding is believed to go on from time to time unpredictably, so shedders are thought to unknowingly start many new cases each year. People who have had the symptoms of herpes (blisters, ulcers) can also transmit the disease by shedding, even if they are not having an attack.

Intercourse is not the only way herpes is transmitted. The disease can pass from your partner to you by any sexual activity where your genitals touch—all kinds of foreplay, and even just cuddling when you're both naked. Oral sex performed on an infected person can result in a genital herpes in your mouth (from their genitals), and having a person infected with oral herpes perform oral sex on you can result in oral herpes sores on your genitals (from their mouth). Oral to genital transmission of the virus is much less common than genital to genital transmission.

What is the difference between oral herpes and genital herpes?

Oral herpes (also called HSV1) and **genital herpes** (HSV2) are caused by different varieties of the same virus. Oral herpes is also what people call canker sores, fever blisters, or cold sores. Generally, oral herpes occurs on or around the mouth and genital herpes on or around the genitals. The two diseases have similar symptoms: Oral herpes causes a sore in or on the mouth and lips that is slow-healing, painful, and contagious and may recur. The symptoms may be milder, with less pain and sores that heal more quickly than on the genitals, but oral herpes, like its genital counterpart, retreats to the nerves and recurs from time to time.

What should I do if I think I might have genital herpes?

If you discover what you think is a herpes blister or ulcer, see your physician *immediately*. Herpes is a painful, serious, long-term disease, easily transmitted, and, though not life-threatening, dangerous to the fetus and newborn if you are pregnant. Don't be embarrassed or let a friend's reassurance overcome your good sense. Only prescription drugs will help. By finding out whether or not you have genital herpes and, if you do, starting treatment early, you can save yourself from worry and—more importantly—a wrong diagnosis. The longer you wait, the more difficult it will be for your doctor to detect the disease before it retreats into the lower genital tract nerves, and the less chance you have to avoid the excruciating pain associated with herpes. You could also, in the meantime, inadvertently pass it on to someone else. Play it safe; see your doctor!

Is there anything I can do before I see a doctor?

Yes. If it's Friday night and your appointment is Monday morning, you can get some relief over the weekend by applying cold, wet towels to your vulva. Since genital herpes is so contagious, *don't* have sex until you've seen the doctor and know you don't have it. Also, be sure to wash your hands thoroughly after touching your genitals; if you touch your eye, you can cause the painful infection pinkeye (conjunctivitis) there, and even your fingers can become infected. You should also avoid sharing washcloths and towels during the initial attack.

Can genital herpes be cured?

Genital herpes is a virus that affects the body cell by cell, entering a healthy cell and taking it over by producing tiny protein invaders that interfere with the cell's normal functions (such as kicking out invaders). No virus is curable, but some—like polio and flu—can be prevented by vaccines that inoculate and protect the body before it is infected. Unfortunately, you can't get vaccinated against herpes. There is no treatment that can completely eradicate the virus from the body. Once it has established itself, the virus will live on in a mostly inactive state. The virus occasionally becomes active, periodically in recurrent attacks.

Though it is not curable, there is a treatment for genital herpes symptoms (described below), which, though it doesn't rid you of the disease, can reduce the frequency, duration, and pain of the recurrent attacks.

How is genital herpes treated? What will my doctor do?

If you develop a blister or ulcer, or if you think you have been exposed, you should go to the doctor. You will have an internal exam, and she will carefully examine your vulva, vagina, and cervix using a **speculum** (a plastic or metal instrument with two long, tongue-shaped blades, which, when inserted into the vagina, spreads its walls in order for the doctor to see the wall of the vagina and the cervix). If the doctor sees bumps, blisters, or sores like those described, she will make a preliminary diagnosis of genital herpes and will also take a sample of fluid from a blister or ulcer, or by swabbing the walls of the vagina or the surface of the cervix. The swabbed fluid is then cultured in a specially prepared test tube at a laboratory and tested to see if the virus is present.

Many women with herpes lesions in the vagina and vulva will develop herpes in the lining of the cervix, too; this is called **herpes cervicitis.** The disease causes microscopic changes—**cervical atypia**—in the cervical cells that can be detected only by a Pap test. Cervicitis can occur during the first and all recurrent attacks. Often, the cervicitis will heal by itself, and the Pap test will then be normal. Sometimes, however, the atypia may persist or recur. Cervical atypia is thought to be a precancerous condition for some women, who may later get cervical cancer.

For this reason, your doctor should always give you a Pap test if herpes is suspected. Follow-up Pap tests after treatment should be given to make sure the cellular abnormalities do not persist. Another good reason for the Pap test is that it is sometimes the only way a woman knows she has contracted herpes and needs treatment and observation should she later become pregnant.

Prior exposure to herpes can be determined from a blood test (which shows antibodies to the disease), but this test won't pinpoint when you got it, how it is affecting your body, or whether it is active or not. The culture test, on the other hand, uses fluid taken directly from a blister or ulcer and will be positive, indicating current infection. The culture will be positive even in asymptomatic shedders if taken from the penis, vulva, vagina, or cervix when shedding is occurring. A culture will be negative when the blisters or ulcers have healed or if an asymptomatic shedder is not shedding at the time the culture is taken.

Your doctor will want to make sure you don't have other diseases that cause ulcers. Traumatic lesions and the syphilis chancre are the two most commonly confused with herpes. The ulcers of traumatic lesions, however, are not as painful, can be traced to a particular injury, and heal more quickly. The syphilis sore is usually deeper and usually painless compared to the herpes sore.

The treatment of herpes is aimed more at relieving the discomfort of the symptoms than curing the disease, which isn't possible. Applying cold, wet towels to your genitals and taking sitz baths (sitting in a warm bath so that your genitals are submerged) using baking soda or drugstore sitz-bath preparations all relieve the pain. You can also take *aspirin* or *Tylenol*. *Tylenol with codeine, Percodan,* or *Percocet* might be prescribed by your doctor if the pain is unbearable and you can't sit comfortably or function normally.

Your doctor will also prescribe *acyclovir* (sold under the brand name of *Zovirax*), a medication that inhibits the virus's ability to reproduce itself. Acyclovir is not a cure and doesn't eradicate the virus from your body, but it slows the virus's growth. The medication can shorten the duration of the initial and recurrent attacks by helping the ulcers heal faster. It also decreases the pain of the lesions but does not prevent transmission of the disease.

In the case of mild recurrent attacks, your doctor may prescribe acyclovir as an ointment to be applied directly to the blisters and ulcers. You will be asked to cover the infected area six times during the day without washing in between.

Acyclovir, which is more effective when taken orally, is prescribed in pill form for an initial attack or severe recurrent attacks. Two-hundred-milligram pills taken five times a day for ten days is the usual dosage for initial attacks, but it is taken for five days for recurrent attacks. Time is important here because acyclovir is most effective if you start using it at the first sign of attack, when the numbness, tingling, or burning sensation preceding the actual blisters is felt. For severe, recurrent herpes, you and your doctor will consider together long-term acyclovir therapy.

If it's not genital herpes, what could cause a blister?

You may confuse a pimple with the blister of an initial herpes attack. Pimples do occasionally occur on the genitals, as they do on the face. But pimples are rounder and tend to occur singly, rather than the many (five to ten) blisters of an initial herpes attack and are much less painful. The herpes blister also tends to be flatter, with the white patches squared off rather than rounded as with a pimple. The herpes ulcer can also be difficult to distinguish from the ulcers caused by other STDs: syphilis, chancroid, and traumatic lesions, all of which are discussed elsewhere in this book. Syphilis ulcers are almost always painless, hard, and deeper than the herpes ulcer, while traumatic ulcers are not nearly as painful and are usually associated with a particular injury or irritation. Chancroid ulcers will not go away unless treated, and though they are painful, they are much less common than herpes. The distinguishing characteristic of herpes is the extremely painful blisters and ulcers it causes.

What happens during a recurrent genital herpes attack? How is it different from the initial attack?

After the initial attack, the herpes virus retreats to the nerves of the lower genital area or tract where it lives on in an inactive state, recurring periodically when triggered by such stresses as lack of sleep, menstruation, poor nutrition, fatigue, or a cold. An attack may even occur spontaneously. Though such stresses are commonly associated with a recurrence, no one knows exactly why people have these repeat attacks. When the virus is reactivated an infected woman may feel itching, numbness, and tingling in her vulva. Though there are no blisters as in the initial attack, an ulcer may appear anywhere on the vulva, anal area, or buttocks. The ulcer may reappear at the initial site of infection or another area. The ulcers are indistinguishable from the initial ulcers, but they are often less painful and heal within two to five days.

Though ninety percent of those initially infected with genital herpes will experience one or more recurrent attacks, over time the frequency and pain of the attacks decrease. There is no way to predict who will get frequent recurrences. Some people will have them once a month, others only several times a year. Most people, even those with frequent recurrences, will have fewer recurrences as years pass.

How can you avoid getting herpes?

The best way to avoid herpes is by not having sexual contact with an infected person. Since you don't always know if someone is infected, use a condom when you do choose to be intimate, especially with a new partner. Condoms provide the only reliable protection against herpes as well as many other STDs. Here are some basic precautions that can help you stay healthy:

- If you or your partner is having an initial attack of herpes (which commonly lasts from two weeks to a month from start to finish), don't have sex—intercourse, oral sex, or anything involving contact with the genitals—even with a condom, as this is the most highly contagious period. Wait until the doctor tells you the sores are completely healed.
- If you or your partner is having a recurrent attack (which usually lasts a week), even if you do use a condom, there is the chance that any ulcers not covered by the condom can still infect you. It's safest to wait.
- If you or your partner has just had an attack, wait until all the ulcers have healed completely before you are intimate. Again, it's best to use a condom during the first few weeks after an attack.
- If your partner has herpes and you don't, and you are planning to get pregnant or are pregnant, condoms should be used throughout your pregnancy.

Are there any side effects to the treatment of herpes with acyclovir?

Although acyclovir appears to be a safe drug, it is a relatively new medication, and little research has been done on it. There is a possibility that it may cause damage to the developing fetus and the newborn, so women who are pregnant or breast-feeding should *not* take it. Some people experience side effects, such as nausea, vomiting, headaches, and diarrhea. For most people, the symptoms are mild enough for them to continue taking the drug anyway. Although there are signs that some varieties of the genital herpes virus may be becoming resistant to acyclovir, it remains the most effective treatment for genital herpes.

Special Risks and Considerations

Though genital herpes is not a life-threatening disease, it remains in a woman's body and can affect her in different ways throughout her life. Two special areas of concern are childbearing and cancer, since special precautions need to be taken during pregnancy and since some kinds of cancer are more common in women who have herpes.

Herpes and Cancer

When the genital herpes virus invades the cells of the cervix, which happens in eight out of ten infected women, it causes inflammation, or **cervicitis.** Though in most cases the cervicitis heals spontaneously as the attack subsides and the ulcers heal, in some women it may not heal, developing over the long term into **atypia** and then **dysplasia.** These are cervical cell conditions in which precancerous changes occur as a result of the inflammation herpes causes. Atypia and dysplasia can be detected with a Pap test. Atypia and dysplasia can eventually become cancer of the cervix. Since studies show that ninety percent of women with cervical cancer have had herpes or other STDs, a woman with herpes should have a Pap test at least once a year. If she has had an abnormal Pap test, this may mean she needs to have more frequent smears. This does not mean that herpes causes cervical cancer directly, but that if you have herpes, your risk of cervical cancer is higher than average.

Though cancer of the vulva is very rare (less than one percent of all genital tract cancers in women are of the vulva), herpes also increases your risk for this type of cancer.

Herpes and Pregnancy

Women who have genital herpes or contract it during pregnancy are more likely to have miscarriages, premature births, and stillbirths. They also run the risk of giving the disease to the child as it passes through the birth canal. Because herpes can cause serious, sometimes life-threatening illness in newborn babies, women with positive herpes cultures at the end of their pregnancies *must* have Caesarean section births to prevent transmission. A woman with herpes should also have cultures taken throughout her pregnancy, more frequently toward the end to be sure the disease is inactive during birth. Women who have herpes on their hands or breasts must also avoid breast-feeding.

If You Have Herpes . . .
- see your doctor.
- have a Pap test annually, or more often as your doctor advises.
- when pregnant, consult with your doctor, who will want to follow your pregnancy closely. See your doctor at the first hint of an attack. Your doctor will want to take herpes cultures during the last weeks of pregnancy to determine the risk of transmission during birth.

GENITAL WARTS

What are genital warts?

Genital warts are a contagious STD caused by infection with HPV, or *human papilloma virus* (also known as condyloma). This is a virus similar to the one that causes plantar or common warts on the hands and feet. Genital warts are treatable, but if they are left untreated, they may grow rapidly. Clinical studies have shown that certain strains of the virus that causes these warts may make cancer of the cervix, vagina, vulva, anus, and penis more likely. Because of this research, genital warts are now treated by physicians as a precancerous condition. Since most people think warts are harmless, there is little public awareness that these growths, when they appear on the genitals, can be dangerous. In fact, genital warts are now the most common viral STD and the second most common STD overall, with at least three million new cases reported each year.

What do genital warts look like?

Since genital warts are caused by a slow-growing virus, it may take three months to two years after infection for a wart to be noticeable. A genital wart is hard to the touch and painless and can be flat or stick out above the surface of the skin and feel fleshy. These warts are flesh-colored or grayish-white and vary greatly in size, shape, and height, though the majority of them are between the size of a pencil point and the size of a dime. When they are raised above the skin, genital warts look like a cauliflower due to their rough, irregular edges. When flat, they might be barely noticeable and just seem like patches of rough skin. Most start out as small, single growths, but if untreated, they can merge and grow rapidly into large masses covering the entire genital area, especially during pregnancy when they are stimulated by high levels of female hormones.

Where do they grow on a woman's genitals?

Genital warts in women usually appear on the vulva, most often on the inner and outer lips, and in or around the anus. Less often, they may be found on the clitoris or around the opening of the urethra. In more than half the cases, women with warts on the vulva also have them internally, in the vagina and cervix, where they may have appeared originally and then spread out. Considering all women with genital warts, about twenty percent have them *only* internally and may never realize they are infected until their doctors tell them or until their partners get them.

Where do they grow on a man's genitals?

In men, warts can appear anywhere on the genitals but occur most often on the head of the penis. Men can also develop warts on the scrotum and anus when warts on the penis spread. An uncircumcised man may also have warts under the foreskin that neither you nor he notices. Anal warts occur frequently in homosexual men since anal intercourse can cause them. Usually, since the male penis and scrotum are completely outside the body, genital warts are easier to notice on a man than they are on a woman.

How do I find out if I have warts, especially internal warts I can't see myself?

Visible, raised warts on the vulva or anus or in the vagina can be seen by your doctor during a thorough gynecological checkup. Flat warts on the cervix and other internal warts are not, however, visible to the naked eye, nor even to the doctor during an examination. These warts are usually discovered after a Pap test that shows abnormalities, or atypia, in the surface cells of the cervix, or during a **colposcopy**. The **colposcope** looks like a telescope with a long, tubular lens that doesn't touch the body as it magnifies the surfaces of the vagina and vulva, revealing small or flat warts not visible to the eye. Colposcopy is performed after an abnormal Pap test or if your doctor suspects a problem with your cervix.

What should I do if I notice a wart on my genitals? Or on my partner?

If you discover what you think is a wart, make an appointment to see your doctor and tell your partner to do the same. You can't, and shouldn't try to, treat warts yourself with over-the-counter treatments because you might seriously damage the sensitive tissue of your genitals. If your partner has a wart on his penis or has had them in the past, both of you need to see a doctor, since you may both have been infected. Remember, warts are slow-growing, and either one of you may have warts that are not yet large enough to be detected. In fact, a recent study showed that seven out of ten male partners of women who had warts also had them. Even colposcopy might not reveal warts at first because the warts are often very small. You should be examined every several months to make sure you have not been infected.

What will my doctor do to remove the warts?

For small warts up to a half inch in size, or when there are only a few on the anus and vulva, many doctors use chemical treatments that burn off or dissolve the wart. Chemical preparations are often applied repeatedly, and one or two applications a week for three to four weeks are often necessary. *Podophyllin,* one chemical treatment, applied *only* by a doctor, usually takes four or five applications until the wart has disappeared. It should be left on for four hours before being washed off with water. Used excessively, Podophyllin can lower blood potassium and bring on seizures, and it should not be used during pregnancy since it may cause damage to the developing baby.

Your doctor can also apply *trichloracetic acid:* it is left on for twelve hours before washing and, like Podophyllin, usually applied several times until the warts have disappeared. Sometimes your doctor may allow you to apply the repeat treatments yourself, under her supervision.

These treatments are for small warts and aren't always the most successful at curing them. A common side effect such treatments cause is a minor irritation of the skin, usually a burning sensation and redness. This irritation usually disappears after several days.

Larger warts of more than one half inch on the vulva and anus and those found internally in the vagina and cervix are treated with any one of the methods that follow. The treatment your doctor chooses depends on both the location and the size of the wart and the method she feels most comfortable using, though all can be equally effective.

Liquid nitrogen is applied directly to the warts and burns them off painlessly. Often, a single treatment is enough.

Cryosurgery uses a sophisticated instrument that destroys the wart by freezing it. Cryosurgery is painless and takes about two minutes.

Heat cautery is an older method that uses electricity to burn off the wart. It is very commonly used and causes only mild pain.

Laser surgery is the newest treatment. It uses a beam of intense light focused on the wart to destroy it. It is used mostly for large warts or multiple warts, if they have been resistant to other treatments. Because it uses an expensive machine, the procedure is done mostly in hospitals. It is also painless.

What can I do to avoid getting warts?

Using condoms is the best preventive measure. Also important is asking your partner if he has ever had warts and, if so, making sure the warts have been treated. If your partner has had warts within the past year or is presently getting treatment, you should have six-month checkups to make sure you haven't caught them and be sure to use a condom.

How do you get warts?

Vaginal or anal intercourse or any other activity that involves frequent genital-to-genital contact with someone who has genital warts can lead to infection. You cannot, however, get warts from oral sex. Common warts on the hands can also be spread to the genitals through touch, but this is rare. Most women get warts from long-term sexual exposure to someone who has them. The longer you are exposed, the greater the risk.

If I had warts in the past and they went away, should I still see my doctor?

Yes, you should have another checkup. Genital warts can disappear spontaneously, but this doesn't mean they're gone forever. In fact, if you had genital warts in the past, your doctor might have told you not to worry and to wait until they disappeared. In the last few years, doctors have discovered that certain strains of genital warts (the human papilloma virus) cause genital and anal cancer. Even with the most sophisticated tests, it is difficult to determine the particular strain causing a specific wart. To avoid this cancer risk, doctors try to treat all warts quickly, with a variety of different methods, until they disappear.

After treatment, be sure to see your doctor for a follow-up exam. The warts could return even without your being exposed to them again. Particles of HPV can lie dormant in the body for weeks or even months and cause repeat attacks.

What else could something that looks like a wart be?

Sometimes **condylomata lata,** or the genital growths of the secondary stage of syphilis, are mistaken for genital warts. Condylomata lata is something only a doctor can diagnose with a blood test. Refer to the section on syphilis for details.

The tiny, white cauliflowerlike growths you may have seen on the head of your partner's penis are often confused with genital warts. About one in one hundred men has these, which have no specific medical name but are commonly called **pearly growths,** and they are due to nothing more than an overgrowth of normal skin cells, like a freckle or a beauty mark. Pearly growths are smaller than warts (about the size of a pencil point), whiter, lighter in color, and occur singly. They usually appear and disappear without treatment. If your partner is not sure about a growth, have him see a doctor to make sure it isn't a wart.

Special Risks and Considerations

Genital Warts and Cancer

Doctors now consider infection of the cervix by human papilloma virus (HPV) the greatest risk factor for cervical cancer because it has been shown that the flat warts found there are frequently caused by cancer-causing strains of HPV. Flat warts are especially dangerous since they may not be visible to the naked eye, even to your doctor during a routine pelvic exam. Pap tests and colposcopy are the only ways to find out you have them. In addition, although cancer of the vulva and vagina is rare, almost all of these cancers occur in women with HPV. For these reasons, HPV and the warts the virus causes are considered a dangerous precancerous condition that should be treated immediately and until the warts are no longer present.

Cancer of the penis and anus also occur more often in men with HPV. Heterosexual women and homosexual men who are the passive partners in anal intercourse get HPV more frequently and are therefore more likely to develop anal cancer, though this is rare.

Genital Warts and Pregnancy

Genital warts during pregnancy are a special concern for women because they can interfere with the birth and be transmitted to the newborn during birth. In pregnancy, stimulated by the high level of female hormones present in the blood, warts can grow large enough to cover the entire vulva. They can become so large that they partially block the birth canal, making Caesarean delivery necessary. Babies born to mothers with genital warts can also develop warts on their vocal cords. For these reasons, it is important to have warts treated before you get pregnant, especially since many of the treatments are either impossible to perform or dangerous to mother and child during pregnancy. Podophyllin, because of its toxic nature, can't be used during pregnancy, and cryosurgery, cautery, or any other method that disturbs the cervix is risky since it might induce labor.

If You Have Genital Warts . . .

- see your doctor immediately for treatment.
- alert your sexual partner(s) to the possibility that they may be infected.
- while you and your partner get treatment, use a condom.
- and are planning a pregnancy or are pregnant, make sure your warts are treated immediately.
- and have already been treated, get periodic checkups to make sure the warts haven't returned. If your partner has had them, you should also have periodic checkups.

CHAPTER TWO

Less Commmon Genital Lesions and Related Conditions

Though today we only hear about the most common STDs—herpes and genital warts—there are other diseases that cause sores, bumps, and other lesions on the surface of the genitals. This chapter covers these less common diseases in some detail because even though they are rare, when they do occur people often mistake them for something else. **Syphilis, chancroid,** and **granuloma inguinale** are all in this category. Although your chances of coming into contact with these diseases are low (granuloma inguinale is a tropical disease, for example), when they do occur they can make you very sick. All of these diseases, however, when accurately diagnosed, can be easily cured with antibiotics.

SYPHILIS

What is syphilis?

Syphilis is an STD caused by the bacterium Treponema pallidum. It has been around for centuries—descriptions of it can even be found in the Bible. It puzzled doctors for many years, becoming known as "the great imitator" because it looked like diseases of the skin, heart, and nervous system. Syphilis is a systemic disease: It first enters the genitals and causes symptoms there but can eventually affect almost every organ system of the body. Caught in the first stage, it is easily curable with antibiotics.

The disease has three distinct stages: the primary stage when the syphilis ulcer, or chancre (pronounced *shan-ker*), appears; a secondary stage during which the disease spreads through the bloodstream to other parts of the body and causes mild symptoms like fatigue, headaches, and rashes; and a final stage in which it infects the heart, blood vessels, and nervous system. If untreated, syphilis attacks major organs and can be fatal. Children born to mothers with syphilis can suffer birth defects or be stillborn. Caught in the first stage with the appearance of the sores, syphilis is easily cured with one dose of penicillin. In the later stages it is much harder to diagnose and treat.

Though syphilis used to be one of the most common STDs in the U.S., the disease declined dramatically from about seventy-three cases per 100,000 people before the introduction of penicillin in the late 1940s to less than four cases per 100,000 in the 1950s.

In the last three decades the incidence of the disease has increased slightly, though for different reasons at different times. In the 1960s and 1970s the increase (mostly in homosexual men) was attributed to changing sexual practices; heterosexuals and homosexuals were more likely to have more sexual partners, and hence more opportunities, if infected, to pass on the disease. Today, with the caution born of AIDS, syphilis in homosexuals has steadily declined, though homosexuals still account for the majority of new cases. In heterosexuals, however, syphilis is on the rise, with many cases traced to prostitutes and people addicted to the form of cocaine known as crack. In New York City alone, the number of syphilis cases has been doubling since 1986. Similar increases have occurred in major cities where drugs and prostitution are prevalent.

Because syphilis is both deadly and highly communicable, by law doctors and testing laboratories must report it to the local health department. Most reporting is done by the laboratories that actually perform the syphilis tests. The infected person is contacted by health officials or a private doctor who will ask for the names of all his or her sexual partners in order to inform those partners of their risk.

What does syphilis look like? What are the symptoms?

After exposure to the disease, it takes from nine to ninety days (usually three weeks) for the first symptom—the syphilis chancre—to appear. The chancre begins as a single, hard, red, painless bump resembling a small pimple that gradually enlarges, wearing away the surface of the skin to become a sore or ulcer that is red and moist, with rough, hardened, often scabbed edges. It varies from the size of a small pimple to an inch in diameter. The formation of the chancre is the first stage of syphilis infection.

The chancre appears at the site of initial contact, usually on the vagina, vulva, cervix, or penis. Homosexual men often get it on the buttocks or anus. It can also appear on the mouth, hands, fingers, or breasts. Along with the chancre, the lymph nodes in the groin may be enlarged, but not painful. The syphilis chancre is highly infectious. Even without treatment, the syphilis chancre heals and completely disappears within four to six weeks. But this does not mean the disease has gone away. At this point, the infected person enters the second stage.

The symptoms of the second stage can appear singly or together and first occur from one week to six months after the chancre has healed. These symptoms vary in severity and are often thought to be due to other medical problems, like a virus or skin disease. After the chancre heals the symptoms become much more varied. The most common symptom is a **rash,** which can appear anywhere on the body but most often occurs on the palms, soles of the feet, back, and chest. The rash consists of small red bumps that are often surrounded by flat areas of redness. The bumps can become enlarged, itchy, and scabby.

Mucous patches—shallow, silvery-gray depressions in the skin surrounded by red edges—occur in about one third of infected people in the secondary stage and are very infectious. They occur on the mucous membranes of the body—on the lips and tongue, inside the mouth, and on the vulva, vagina, and penis.

Condyloma lata—moist, pink cauliflowerlike growths that can become huge masses—may also appear on the genital skin, the vulva, at the base of the penis, and on the groin where the upper thigh meets the genitals. Sometimes such growths also occur under the arms and beneath the breasts. They are also very infectious.

Common symptoms that appear in some but not all of those infected include fever, headache, weight loss, fatigue, loss of appetite, and hair loss in patches on the head. Painless swelling of the lymph glands under the arms, beneath the chin, and elsewhere on the body is also common. The symptoms of the second stage usually last for several months but may come and go for several years. During this time the infected person is very contagious, especially because of the bacteria present in the rashes and lesions.

It is very difficult to diagnose syphilis in the second stage because many of the symptoms are elusive and similar to those of more common, less dangerous diseases. The general symptoms and rashes of secondary syphilis are often misdiagnosed as other disorders, such as simple viral infections, allergic reactions, and skin conditions. Unfortunately, if syphilis is not diagnosed in the second stage, it is often not recognized at all.

After the second-stage symptoms disappear, the

disease is said to be "latent" or resting, though the infection is still present. During the latent stage there may be no ongoing symptoms, but the individual may relapse and experience second stage symptoms again and again—most often within two years and less often after that. Throughout this secondary stage the infected person is only contagious when rashes or lesions are present. The latent stage can last a lifetime.

About one third of all untreated people who pass through the second and latent stages will develop third stage or **tertiary syphilis,** in which the nervous system and cardiovascular system (heart and blood vessels) are affected. Tertiary syphilis usually occurs from ten to twenty years after the secondary stage. It can affect the brain and spinal cord, damaging nerves that control position and balance of the body; cause difficulty in walking; and affect bladder control. Blindness, psychosis, and loss of sensation may occur, as well as many other complications. In the cardiovascular system syphilis can cause abnormalities of the heart valves and blood vessels, sometimes leading to heart murmurs, heart failure, or the rupture of blood vessels. Complications arising from tertiary syphilis can be fatal.

How do you get syphilis?

Syphilis is transmitted by contact with an infectious syphilis lesion—chancre, condyloma lata, or mucous patch—during vaginal or anal intercourse, or by having oral sex with a person who has the chancre, which is highly contagious. You can get it from a person in the second stage from any contact with the condyloma lata and mucous patches or any other skin lesions or rashes, which are all highly infectious. The disease enters the body at the site of contact with the chancre, condyloma lata, or mucous patch so that performing oral sex on a man who has the sore on his penis may result in a sore on the partner's lips and inside the mouth, and fondling or masturbating one's partner can result in sores on the fingers or breasts. Because the syphilis chancre may appear on the vagina and is painless, many women never know they have it until it is discovered during a routine gynecological exam. This is another good reason to have such an exam once a year, especially if you think, for any reason, that you might have been exposed to an STD. The blood of an infected person is also infectious, but all blood banks test for syphilis and other STDs. Catching syphilis from a blood transfusion is extremely rare.

How will my doctor know I have syphilis?

If you think you may have been exposed sometime in the past, have your doctor give you a syphilis blood test, which will always show whether or not you have the disease. Syphilis can also be diagnosed, but not reliably, in the secondary stage with the appearance of the condyloma lata or any other secondary-stage symptom.

Your doctor will look for the chancre, condyloma lata, and mucous patches and check your lymph nodes for swelling. She may take a sample of a chancre, if present, and send it to a lab for **dark field microscopic examination,** which reliably shows the syphilis bacteria. Your doctor will always take a blood sample for testing, though which test she uses will depend on how long ago you think you were exposed and whether or not you have the chancre. Testing the blood is the most reliable way to diagnose syphilis.

The two most commonly used tests are called *VDRL* and *FTA;* both measure antibodies produced by the body six to seven weeks after exposure or infection. FTA is most reliable in diagnosing syphilis in the primary stage when the chancre is present or when someone suspects he/she may have been exposed but doesn't yet have the chancre. VDRL is used when the person is believed to have passed into the secondary stage because it is not highly reliable for people in the first stage who only have the chancre.

Both tests have limitations and aren't reliable in certain cases. Drug addicts, pregnant women, and people with certain immune disorders (like lupus), for example, are sometimes shown by VDRL to have syphilis when they actually do not have it. Because the tests aren't one hundred percent reliable, if you think you have syphilis but had a negative test you should have another test after six weeks.

After treatment the VDRL test usually becomes negative while the FTA test of an infected person usually remains positive throughout his or her life. For this reason, VDRL is used during treatment to see if the treatment is effective, and it is used after treatment as a check that the disease has been eradicated from the body.

How is syphilis treated? What exactly will my doctor do?

After diagnosis, syphilis in every stage can be completely cured, usually by a single dose of long-acting penicillin, *benzathine penicillin G*, given by injection of a dose of 2.4 million units into the muscle. Shorter-acting penicillins like *penicillin V, procaine penicillin,* and *ampicillin* are only effective against syphilis contracted within ten days—which is often hard to determine. For those allergic to penicillin, your doctor will prescribe *tetracycline*, 500 milligrams taken four times daily by mouth for fifteen days. Penicillin side effects are rare, but the drug can cause rashes and hives.

Fever, chills, and muscle aches can occur in up to half of those with first stage syphilis and ninety percent of those in the second stage, not as a side effect but as a result of treatment. Your doctor will warn you of this. This strong reaction, while not completely understood, is probably the result of a disturbance of the immune balance in the body as the antibiotic attacks the disease.

If you have had syphilis for more than a year, or if you show symptoms that syphilis may have invaded the nervous system, your doctor may advise a **spinal tap.** In this procedure, a small amount of fluid is drawn from the spinal cord under local anesthesia and then tested for syphilis. If there are signs of nervous system infection or indications that syphilis has been present in the body for more than one year, the disease is treated with higher doses (six to nine million units) of longer-acting penicillin. If damage to the nervous system has already occurred, the treatment does not reverse it but often can prevent further symptoms.

In all cases, your partner should be treated at the same time that you are. You should not have sex until after a blood test has shown that you no longer have the disease. *You and your partner both need to be tested again after treatment*. Such tests should be given three, six, and twelve months after treatment to ensure the cure was total. Your doctor may recommend a slightly different schedule of retesting. Occasionally, treatment will need to be repeated.

If the sore is not syphilis, what else could it be?

Traumatic ulcers caused by injury to the genitals like a zipper that pinches your skin, or chafed red patches from vigorous sex or use of a vibrator, don't usually resemble the syphilis sore. They heal very quickly in several days and don't have the punched-out shape of the chancre. The sores from **genital herpes** form more than one ulcer, are shallow, and are extremely painful. Since syphilis chancres usually occur singly, are punched out, and are painless, the two are easy to distinguish. Also, the lymph node enlargement in herpes is painful, while in syphilis it is not. Symptoms of **chancroid,** which is much rarer, include a painful ulcer that is soft, not hard as in syphilis, and occurs only on the genitals, most often in groups. **Granuloma inguinale,** even rarer than syphilis, has as a symptom a painless plaque (an irregularly shaped raised area of open skin rising above the surface of normal skin) and tends to cause a much greater enlargement of the groin lymph nodes, which are visibly swollen and bulge out of the groin.

What can I do to avoid getting syphilis? To avoid giving it to someone else?

Since syphilis is transmitted during intimate sexual contact, you should always use a condom. Look out for any unusual sores, blisters, or bumps on your partner's lips and mouth, penis, and genital area. If he or she has a sore on the lips, mouth, or tongue, you should avoid all sexual contact until it has been checked by a doctor. If you think you have syphilis, you should avoid all sexual activity until you've seen your doctor, especially if you have a sore, which is highly contagious. You should also, if the diagnosis is syphilis, tell your partner that he may have been infected and to see a doctor immediately.

Prostitutes, IV drug users, and homosexual men have a much higher incidence of syphilis than the general population.

Special Risks and Considerations

Syphilis and Pregnancy

Since syphilis can cross through the placenta or birth sac, an infected woman can pass it on to her unborn child in the uterus. A woman who has had untreated syphilis for a year has an eighty to ninety-five percent risk of passing it on to her newborn. Even in the latent stage, up to four years after exposure, there is still a seventy percent chance of infecting the fetus. During pregnancy, syphilis infection can cause miscarriage and, more commonly, stillbirth. Birth defects and even blindness can occur. Infants born to infected mothers may develop rashes and skin lesions like the infected adult and later develop bone and liver diseases and anemia. Most infants with syphilis do not die but later suffer from eye, joint, and neurological problems. Death, when it does occur, happens in the first few months of life from bleeding into the lungs, pneumonia, or liver disease. These are all good reasons why, if you are pregnant or planning to get pregnant, you should be tested for syphilis.

Syphilis and Other Diseases

An open area of skin like the syphilis chancre or mucous patch invites invasion by bacteria and viruses. People with syphilis, in fact, have a much higher incidence of other STDs like gonorrhea and herpes and may run a greater risk of contracting AIDS for the same reason.

If you think you have syphilis . . .

- see your doctor immediately.
- don't have any form of sex; you may be highly contagious.
- wait for the results of your blood test, even if your doctor has good reason to suspect syphilis, before informing your partner. The test will reliably tell you if you have the disease, and that way you can avoid unduly alarming others.

CHANCROID

What is chancroid?

Chancroid is a nonfatal tropical STD with only
one thousand cases seen a year in the U.S., those
reported mostly in merchant seamen or soldiers recently returned from Southeast Asia, Africa, and Central America, where the disease is more common.
There have, however, been recent localized out-
breaks—in California in 1983 there were 923 cases
traced to local prostitutes. Overall, chancroid is very
rare in women, and even in tropical countries where
the disease is more common the majority of infected
women are prostitutes.

What does chancroid look like? What are the symptoms?

Chancroid is caused by Hemophilus ducreyi bacteria and is transmitted through vaginal or anal
intercourse. Three to five days after infection small red
bumps form, singly or in groups, on the labia or around
the anus in women, and anywhere on the penis in men.
Two to three days later the bump breaks down into an
ulcer or sore on the surface of the skin. The sores vary
from a pencil point to a dime in size. They have ragged
edges and blend in with the surrounding skin. The
ulcer is soft, covered with a thin layer of pus, and
painful. The lymph nodes in the groin swell painfully. If
untreated, the ulcer will not heal, and the lymph nodes

in the groin will become very swollen and filled with pus.

How is chancroid treated? What will my doctor do?

After examining your genitals the doctor will take a culture of the infection by swabbing the sore. After the sample of disease organism is grown in a culture, a lab test will show whether or not it is chancroid. If the test is positive, the chancroid will be quickly and easily cured with antibiotics. Your doctor will usually prescribe either *erythromycin* (trade name, Emycin) or *trimethoprim sulfamethoxazole* (Bactrim/Septra). Erythromycin is one of the most commonly prescribed antibiotics; its common side effects include nausea, vomiting, and diarrhea. Less commonly, liver damage may occur.

What else could a sore be?

An ulcer or sore might be confused with **syphilis, granuloma inguinale,** or **herpes.** See the syphilis section for a summary of these diseases' characteristics. The distinguishing characteristics of chancroid are soft, shallow sores and swollen lymph nodes, and the fact that the sore does not heal without treatment.

What should I do if I think I have chancroid?

You can take aspirin or Tylenol for temporary pain relief. You should see your doctor as soon as possible.

Don't have sex until you've consulted your doctor, and tell your partner to see a doctor. Your doctor will have to use lab tests to make an accurate diagnosis.

How can I avoid getting chancroid?

Since it is transmitted through vaginal or anal intercourse, use a condom and make sure your partner is healthy. Be especially careful if you or your partner are traveling in areas where chancroid is common and are sexually active there.

GRANULOMA INGUINALE

What is granuloma inguinale?

Granuloma inguinale, also called Donovanosis, is another extremely rare STD much more prevalent in tropical or undeveloped countries than in the United States, where only one hundred cases a year are reported. Caused by the bacterium Calymatobacterium granulomatosis, this disease is not fatal but, if untreated, can cause scarring of the genital, anal, and groin areas over time.

What does granuloma inguinale look like? How do you get it?

Because it is so rare, little is known about granuloma inguinale. It is thought that many contacts involving anal or vaginal intercourse are necessary for transmission to occur. Several weeks to months after exposure, a bump appears underneath the skin of the vulva, anywhere on the penis, or near the anus. The skin over the bump erodes within several days, creating a painless, red, slightly raised, moist sore that is covered with an unpleasant-smelling residue.

The lymph nodes in the groin also swell in most cases. The swelling can be great, with the lymph nodes sticking out in the groin area like golf balls under the skin. Sometimes the skin over the enlarged lymph nodes will wear away, looking like yellow-white masses in the V of the groin. Eventually, scars form over the lymph nodes.

How will my doctor diagnose and treat it?

If you haven't lived or traveled extensively in Third World countries or had intimate contact with someone who has, what you have is probably not granuloma inguinale. Your doctor will ask about this and take a biopsy, or tissue sample, for microscopic examination. If it's not granuloma inguinale, it could be chancroid or syphilis. A chancroid symptom is a painful sore that is not raised like the plaque of granuloma, and the syphilis chancre heals by itself in several weeks.

Treatment of granuloma inguinale is uncomplicated. Your doctor will prescribe any of a variety of antibiotics.

LYMPHOGRANULOMA VENEREUM (LGV)

What is LGV?

Caused by one strain of the bacterium Chlamydia trachomatis, **LGV** is an STD common in tropical, undeveloped countries, but even rarer than **granuloma inguinale** in the United States. It is not a fatal disease, but over the long term it can cause scarring and deformity of the groin area.

How do I know I have it? What are the symptoms?

Three days to three weeks after having vaginal intercourse with an infected partner, a small, pimple-sized, usually painless ulcer or sore develops on the penis or vulva. It usually heals, unnoticed, in one week. The infection, however, spreads during this time to the lymph nodes of the groin, causing them to swell extensively and painfully. The skin over the lymph nodes becomes thin and scarred (looking matted, uneven, or stretched), and pus may drain through the skin from the lymph nodes. When the lymph nodes swell and scar from the infection they cease to perform their normal function of draining fluid from the groin area. As a result, lymph node scarring can cause the penis or vulva to swell with fluid.

How is it treated? What will my doctor do?

The doctor will make sure it is LGV by using a needle to draw pus from the swollen lymph nodes and then having a laboratory culture or grow the bacterium and identify it. After diagnosis the doctor will prescribe *tetracycline*.

If it's not LGV, what else could it be?

LGV is distinguished by the swelling and infection of the lymph nodes, though it does cause an ulcer, as do many other STDs. LGV might be confused with syphilis, granuloma inguinale, genital herpes, or chancroid; see the syphilis section for the characteristics of these diseases.

BARTHOLIN'S GLAND INFECTIONS

The **Bartholin's glands** are two pea-sized glands on either side of the opening of the vagina that produce fluid to lubricate the vagina when the body is sexually aroused. You can't see them because they're beneath the skin, delivering the fluid they produce to the surface through narrow ducts. Because the ducts are so narrow, they can become clogged by their own normal secretions, or by fecal material from the nearby anus, and sometimes by bacteria like gonorrhea or mycoplasma. When this happens the glands become infected, swelling the labia and causing acute pain. The blocked duct and gland together are referred to as a **Bartholin's cyst.**

Bartholin's gland infection (BGI) is most often caused by infection from the bacteria found normally in human feces. It is only an STD when caused by gonorrhea or mycoplasma. Fecal bacteria can cause infection when they reach the vulva when a woman wipes toward the vulva rather than away from it. They can sometimes reach the vulva in other ways (on clothes, during sex, or by themselves) simply because the anus is nearby.

Some women are born with narrow Bartholin's ducts, and often with one duct narrower than the other. It is the narrower side that is prone to infection. In my experience, about one in one hundred women will have BGI once. Once you get it, however, you're more likely to get it in the same side again. Unfortunately, after repeated BGIs the ducts become scarred and even narrower and hence prone to further infection.

How do I know if I have a Bartholin's gland infection?

When the Bartholin's glands become blocked with fluid, they become infected. The infection causes swelling, which may not be noticeable to you. If the infection persists, however, the swelling causes the part of the vulva on the side of the infection to become hugely swollen, a lump you will certainly notice. Other symptoms are labia that look distorted in shape (the swelling makes one side look huge), are red, and feel extremely tender and hot to the touch. If the infection persists and you still haven't sought treatment, an abscess—a cavity the size of a golfball filled with pus—can form beneath the skin of the vulva, making sitting and even standing uncomfortable. Women with these infections may also have trouble urinating. If untreated, the infection can spread to surrounding areas and might even enter the bloodstream, causing symptoms like fever and chills.

How will my doctor treat the infection?

If the infection is mild and the swelling minimal, your doctor will prescribe antibiotics to be taken orally. *Keflex* (cephalexin), which is effective against a wide variety of the bacteria that may have caused the infection, is a common choice; 250 milligrams taken four times a day for at least one week is the usual prescription. Most people can take Keflex with no side effects, but others may experience diarrhea or an allergic rash. Your doctor may prescribe other antibiotics.

For infections that are more severe, the doctor may make a small incision into the infected area and drain the pus from it. This simple procedure can be performed in the office using a **local anesthetic** given by injection. She will also take a sample of the fluid, which will be sent to a lab to test for the presence of any STDs (like the gonorrhea mentioned earlier) that may have caused the infection in the first place. Your doctor may also recommend sitz baths to help relieve pain and swelling.

In severe cases, when an abscess has formed, a short hospital stay may be required both because the pain is excruciating and because the antibiotics re-

quired to combat the infection need to be given intra-
venously (through an IV needle inserted into a vein in
the arm). Sometimes a surgical procedure called **marsupialization** is performed, in which part of the duct
wall is removed and the incision sewn so that the gland
empties directly into the vagina. This means that the
duct is bypassed completely, making further infection
unlikely.

How can I avoid Bartholin's gland infections?

Unfortunately, there is no easy way to prevent
infection except to practice good personal hygiene and
wipe carefully from front to back after bowel movements, avoiding contact of fecal matter with the genital
area.

MOLLUSCUM CONTAGIOSUM

What is molluscum contagiosum?

Sometimes called "the pox," **molluscum contagiosum** is a viral infection of the skin that poses no
real health threat but does cause itching and is contagious. It can be transmitted by any close skin-to-skin
contact as well as intimate sexual contact, and through
shared clothing or towels. It occurs in places where
many people share close quarters—military barracks,
dormitories, and beach houses, for example. It is easy
to treat and not serious.

What does the pox look like?

Within a few weeks of exposure to the virus, dome-shaped white or flesh-colored bumps appear on the skin of the genitals, the groin, and sometimes the abdomen and chest. These bumps have small "belly-button"-like depressions on their surfaces and may feel itchy. They might be mistaken for pimples, except that they are usually bigger and often occur in large numbers. The bumps are painless and waxy, containing a smooth, white, cheeselike substance rather than pus. If you notice such bumps, see your doctor. The infection is contagious and uncomfortable. You should also tell your partner that you have it and make sure he hasn't been infected, too.

What is the treatment?

The doctor will scrape a sample of the white substance from a bump and examine it under a microscope. If it is indeed pox, she will see "molluscum" bodies, which are nothing more than clumps of dead skin cells containing particles of the virus. After this painless procedure she will then apply *Podophyllin* or *Trichloracetic acid* to the bumps with a cotton-tipped swab. The pox may also be treated with *liquid nitrogen*. Often, several visits will be necessary before the condition is cleared up. Although the pox usually disappears by itself after six months to a year, it is best to have it treated to prevent its spread and the discomfort it can cause you and others.

CRABS AND SCABIES

Crabs (pubic lice) and scabies are tiny parasitic insects that cannot live anywhere but on the human body. When a person has crabs or scabies he or she is said to be "infested," rather than "infected," as with a bacterium or virus. Crabs and scabies are most common among people who live in crowded conditions without access to good sanitation. Generally the condition is uncommon, especially when compared to such STDs as chlamydia, herpes, or genital warts. Having crabs or scabies is an aggravating, rather than a serious, problem, and the treatment is simple and effective. Many people think crabs are something only people with poor hygiene can get. But since casual contact with an infested person most often results in transmission, you can get them no matter how "clean" you are or what your life-style is.

Pubic Lice or Crabs

What are crabs?

Phthirus pubis, or crabs, are tiny insects that, unlike "head" lice or "body" lice, live only in the pubic hair. Up close they look very much like the crabs that live in the ocean, with four legs like crab claws that grip the pubic hair tightly, though they are only about one tenth of an inch in size. From more than a foot away, however, they may look like tiny brown specks or freckles.

How do I know I have crabs?

You may not know you have crabs until about a month after someone's passed them on to you, when they are numerous enough so that the irritation caused by their bites causes itching. Several weeks after you've been infested you can actually see them—tiny brown spots that move through your pubic hair. At that point most people usually see a doctor.

How do you get rid of crabs?

If your doctor finds crabs, she will prescribe *gamma benzene hexachloride,* known by the brand names *Kwell* and *Lindane.* Applied as a lotion, cream, or shampoo, Kwell kills the insect and its eggs. Before application, wash your whole body with mild soap and dry off. The cream or lotion is applied directly to the pubic hair and skin surrounding the genitals and left on for twelve hours overnight. Usually, one treatment is effective. After the time is up, wash again thoroughly, then see your doctor again to make sure you're rid of the insects. Though Kwell is generally safe for adults, if used excessively it can cause skin irritation. Kwell should not be used by pregnant women or children under the age of ten since it can cause seizures in newborns and young children. In these cases, your doctor may recommend any of several over-the-counter treatments that are not as strong or effective as Kwell. These include *A 200 Pyrinate, Triple X,* and *Rid,* all of which should be used only as directed by your doctor.

Though getting crabs isn't pleasant and you may feel a little embarrassed, the longer you wait for treatment, the more discomfort you will feel. You also run the risk of passing it on to others. Vigorous scrubbing, shaving the pubic hair, and using harsh soaps won't help. Crabs cement their eggs to the skin with a very strong glue, leaving the next generation to plague you. You can spread them to your armpits, facial hair, and even your eyebrows and lashes when you try to remove them yourself. So if you think you have crabs, don't try to treat them yourself. See your doctor!

How do you get crabs?

Crabs are transmitted from person to person most often through any intimate sexual contact when one person's pubic hair comes into contact with another's, allowing the crabs to crawl from one person to the other. Crabs may also infest clothing, towels, bed-sheets, and blankets and are passed on when these items are shared. You can also, believe it or not, get them from a toilet seat—one of the rare instances in which the old wives' tale has some truth to it!

There is no especially effective preventive measure to avoid getting crabs. You can, however, make sure a new partner is clean and isn't itching, and avoid sharing towels or clothes.

If you have crabs . . .

- see your doctor for treatment.
- and you're pregnant or have children under ten who have them, *don't* use Kwell. Ask your doctor for alternative treatments.
- inform all those with whom you've had intimate contact or shared personal items.

- launder in hot water or dry clean all sheets, towels, clothes, blankets, etc.

Scabies

What are scabies?

Scabies is a skin disease caused by sarcoptes scabei, or the itch mite, a microscopic insect that burrows into your skin to live and lay eggs. Unlike crabs, scabies can occur anywhere on the body; the underside of the wrist and between the fingers are common sites. Elsewhere on the body, however, scabies attacks men and women differently. In men it is often found on the skin of the penis, while in women it appears on the breasts, nipples, abdomen, and on the bottom of the buttocks, but not in the pubic area. If untreated, some cases of scabies can last for years.

How do you get scabies?

You are most likely to get scabies, like crabs, from an infested person by having intimate sexual contact in which your skin touches his. Also like crabs, scabies can infest clothes, bedding, and towels. Close sexual contact is not necessary to transmit it, and even sharing a bed with an infested person, holding hands, and hugging can pass it on. Sometimes whole households get scabies, as can roommates who live in close quarters or share personal belongings.

How do you know you have scabies?

It takes at least a month after transmission before a person discovers he or she has scabies, usually from the intense itch the burrowing mites cause, especially at night or after a shower, when the skin is warmer than usual. The only sign of the mites is the tiny red dots, like pinpricks, where they entered the skin. Scratching, however, destroys these marks, as does the red rash that often develops from allergy to the mites. The rash is a series of red bumps covering up to several inches of skin that often looks like scabbed pimples after being scratched intensely. The itching also makes the rash worse, creating areas of red, irritated skin that can in turn become infected by bacteria.

How is scabies treated?

You cannot treat scabies yourself and should see your doctor if you think you have the symptoms (remember that scabies doesn't affect the pubic area in women). Your doctor will first make sure it isn't crabs, acne, or any other skin disease with similar symptoms such as an allergic reaction. Vigorous scrubbing, long showers, and strong soaps will only irritate your skin further and make you itch more.

To confirm a diagnosis of scabies, the doctor will use a sterile needle or scalpel blade to extract a mite from its burrow for identification under a microscope. Once identified, the most common treatment, as with crabs, is *Kwell*. First, wash thoroughly with mild soap and gently towel dry. Then the entire body below the chin is covered with Kwell, which is left on overnight for twelve hours before another washing. Often more than one treatment is necessary, and you should check with your doctor after each treatment to be sure the mites have been eradicated.

If you are pregnant or have children under ten who are infested, you can use *benzyl benzoate* in a twenty-five percent solution instead of Kwell, or *crotamiton* (brand name, *Eurax*), which is applied overnight for two nights. Both of these medications should be used only under your doctor's supervision.

To prevent family members or those sharing living space from passing scabies back and forth, the whole household should be treated at the same time.

How do you avoid getting crabs and scabies?

If you don't share clothes or bedding, especially when living in close quarters like a beach house or dormitory, then you can usually be sure you won't get crabs or scabies even if someone else has them. Since they both can be transmitted through sex, too, don't be intimate with an infested person.

If you have scabies . . .
- see your doctor for immediate treatment.
- tell all sexual partners, or those with whom you come into close contact, to see a doctor.
- and you're pregnant or have infested children under ten, see your doctor, who will provide alternatives to treatment with Kwell.

II
Vaginitis and Urinary Tract Infections (UTIs)

Two of the most common medical conditions women suffer are **vaginitis** and **urinary tract infections (UTIs)**. Most women will have both at least once in their lives, and both can also be chronic, coming and going in some women for a period of years. Though neither is fatal, or even serious in most cases, both are uncomfortable and unpleasant.

Vaginitis and UTIs can be sexually transmitted or brought on by the irritation of sexual intercourse. Both conditions occur when the normal environment of the vulva and vagina is disturbed by common bacteria. In the next sections you will learn how to make getting either one less likely, and how to recognize each condition and how your doctor will treat them.

CHAPTER THREE

Vaginitis

In childbirth, sexual intercourse, and menstruation, the vagina serves as a passageway between the inner reproductive organs and the outside world. While acting as a passageway, the vagina also acts as a barrier—to bacteria, to fecal matter from around the anus, and to other sources of infection outside the body. The constant secretions of the vagina and cervix, which normally vary in consistency, amount, and color with the menstrual cycle, ward off infection and help avoid irritation through lubrication. Just as saliva cleanses, fights infection, and regulates the environment of the mouth, vaginal secretions help maintain the delicate balance between the inside and outside world in the vagina.

The Normal Vagina

Maintaining this balance is not an easy task. The vagina, with its opening so near the anus and urethra, is vulnerable to attack from bacteria that are found normally in feces. These bacteria can easily get into the vagina during such commonplace activities as wiping after a bowel movement.

To protect itself, the vagina makes its own special kind of bacteria, called lactobacilli. Lactobacilli break down the sugar stored in the lining of the vagina into an acid, which makes the environment extremely difficult for alkaline-loving bacteria to live in. In addition to the lactobacilli, there are also normally present in the vagina such organisms as the yeast candida and the bacteria streptococcus and staphylococcus. These "native" organisms, when maintained in a balance, pose no threat of infection and, in fact, help ward off other infectious invaders. When the balance is disturbed, however, one of them (usually yeast) may get the upper hand and cause an infection.

The menstrual cycle plays an important role in determining the vaginal environment. In the menstrual cycle's first stage (which actually begins during the menstrual period), the body makes estrogen, which builds up the vaginal epithelium, or lining. During these two weeks women may experience an "estrogen discharge" in which some of those cells in the lining are shed, causing a mucous discharge that is clear with whitish flecks. Estrogen prepares the reproductive system for ovulation, and fourteen days after the end of the last period the estrogen discharge stops.

At this point progesterone, the other main female hormone, triggers ovulation—the release of an egg from the ovary. The cervix produces secretions that are thin, clear, and elastic—properties that help sperm penetration. Normal vaginal secretions are usually clear, stringy, thin, and odorless.

The menstrual cycle also affects the acidity of the vaginal environment and thus the bacteria that are normally found there. During the early weeks, the acidity of the vagina is high due to the estrogen release, creating an unfavorable environment for bacterial growth. At ovulation, however, estrogen release stops, and the cervix begins to secrete large amounts of alkaline mucus, lowering the acidity and thus decreasing the protection from infection an acid environment provides.

Since an alkaline environment favors bacterial growth, vaginal infections commonly occur during the third and fourth weeks of the cycle. Menstrual fluid is also quite alkaline, and during menstruation all the bacteria that are in balance are flushed out. With an alkaline environment, the native yeast or bacteria from the outside can establish themselves and cause an infection just before and during menstruation.

STD-caused vaginitis can occur at any time, though the symptoms tend to worsen with menstruation.

What is vaginitis?

Vaginitis means literally "inflammation of the vagina," and it occurs when the delicate balance of the vagina is upset by a sexually transmitted infection like **gardnerella** or **trichomonas;** by a frequently occurring microorganism like **yeast;** by chemical substances in douches and contraceptive foams and jellies that irritate the vagina; and sometimes just by overuse of "feminine hygiene" products or use of old antibiotic medication to treat what are actually normal secretions.

What causes sexually transmitted vaginitis, and how is it transmitted?

The three most common causes of vaginitis—gardnerella, trichomonas, and yeast—can all be sexually transmitted. Gardnerella is almost always sexually transmitted and trichomonas is usually sexually transmitted, while yeast vaginitis is only rarely sexually transmitted and so is not considered an STD.

Gardnerella

Gardnerella is now believed to cause at least half of all cases of vaginitis. A bacterium known as hemophilus vaginalis or corynebacterium vaginale, gardnerella is transmitted through sexual intercourse with a man who carries the bacteria in the urethra of his penis. When exposed to the vagina, gardnerella interacts with certain other naturally occurring bacteria (called "anaerobic" because they don't need oxygen to grow) to produce the symptoms of vaginitis. Many men and women have gardnerella in their genitals yet never have any symptoms. The organism is found more often in people with multiple sex partners, women who use IUDs, and women who have cervicitis.

Trichomonas

Trichomonas vaginitis accounts for nearly a quarter of all vaginal infections. A protozoon (a single-cell organism like an amoeba), trichomonas has a pear-shaped body and several sets of antennalike flagella or tails that make it very mobile and very infectious. It is thought that trichomonas causes vaginitis by producing a substance that irritates the vaginal lining. Some men and women commonly have trichomonas protozoa in their genitals but have no symptoms of discharge or itching. Sometimes it turns up on a routine Pap test. Some may develop symptoms later or pass it on to their partners.

Sexual intercourse and other activities in which vaginal or penile fluids from an infected person come into contact with your genitals (even via the fingers) can transmit trichomonas. Though mostly transmitted through such intimate contact, this organism can live outside the body for several hours, which means you can also get it from sharing towels, underwear, bathing suits, douching equipment, or vibrators with an infected person. Though unlikely, it is possible you could be exposed by using a hot tub, pool, or toilet seat used recently by an infected person.

Yeast

Yeast-related vaginitis is caused by a fungus called monilia or candida that is responsible for about one quarter of vaginitis infections. Not usually sexually transmitted, yeast is found throughout the environment and can normally exist in the body. Yeast is even found normally in the vagina in thirty percent of all women (though many will never develop symptoms of infection from it) and in the intestinal tracts of healthy men and women. It is only when the balance is upset—in women who take antibiotics frequently, who are pregnant, who take birth control pills, or who have **diabetes mellitus** (sugar diabetes)—that the yeast flourishes, causing inflammation of the vagina and vulva. In pregnancy (which causes high hormone levels) and diabetes mellitus (which causes high blood sugar levels), for example, the vaginal environment becomes highly acidic, a condition favorable to yeast growth. Other yeast-promoting factors include taking steroid medications like prednisone (used to treat conditions like rheumatoid arthritis, asthma, and lupus), which suppress the immune system. Yeast vaginitis is not often sexually transmitted for two reasons. First, men don't usually get it because the penis is outside the body, and therefore not a good environment for yeast growth; and second, since men very rarely contract a yeast infection of the penis from an infected woman, they are much less likely to pass it on to another woman. For unknown reasons, some women are more prone than others to bout after bout of yeast-related vaginitis.

How do I know I have a vaginal infection or vaginitis?

Vaginal discharge (excessive fluid or moisture leaking from the vagina) is the most frequent symptom. Itching of the vulva, burning when urinating, painful sexual intercourse, and vaginal bleeding are also symptoms of vaginal infection and vaginitis. Though vaginal discharge is the most frequent symptom, you may have any or all symptoms, and they may vary in severity.

Any noticeable change in the secretions of the vagina is known as a vaginal discharge. As explained earlier, normal secretions occur all the time and change in consistency and appearance with the menstrual cycle.

In gardnerella vaginitis, the discharge is gray-white, watery, and heavy. Its smell is distinctive, foul, sour, and fishy. Trichomonas discharge is yellow-green and foamy or bubbly, and it often occurs at the beginning of your period. Its odor is unpleasant, but not as strong as gardnerella. Yeast vaginitis doesn't always produce a discharge. When it does the fluid is thick, white, pasty, and sticky. If heavy, it can have whitish clumps that look like cottage cheese and smell cheesy or sweet, unlike either gardnerella or trichomonas.

Itchiness from irritation of the vulva (the vagina has few nerve endings, and thus you can't feel superficial pain there) is the most frequent symptom of yeast infections. Gardnerella does not cause itchiness but trichomonas does.

Yeast infections cause an intense itch, as well as soreness and a burning or stinging feeling in the vulva, which looks red and dry. The itch and irritation can also spread to your upper thighs and anus. Sometimes yeast infections also cause a rash to spread from the vulva to the upper thighs. The rash is like that which occurs on the dry, reddened, irritated areas of the vulva. Often, a severe rash is actually an allergic reaction to the yeast. The skin looks reddened and is covered with flat or slightly raised patches of rash that itch and burn. If the rash gets worse, the skin becomes covered with raised, pimply patches that ooze fluid. It can be very sore and itchy.

Trichomonas usually causes itching only when the discharge is heavy and may also involve soreness and a burning sensation in the vulva. The itch and irritation of this infection can be particularly severe.

Dysuria, a burning sensation when you urinate, is a much less common symptom of vaginitis, but it can occur when the vulvar swelling involves the urethral opening. This symptom occurs mostly with yeast or trichomonas infections. If you feel burning on urination and there is no discharge and no vulvar itching, you could have a urinary tract infection (see UTI section) and not vaginitis.

Dyspareunia, painful sexual intercourse, usually occurs in vaginitis only when the symptoms described above are also present, since it is caused by the inflammation of the lining of the vagina and vulva. If sexual intercourse is painful but you have no other symptoms of a vaginal infection, this could indicate a problem more serious than vaginitis, such as cervical infection, Bartholin's cyst, or another problem in your cervix, uterus, or tubes.

Vaginal bleeding is also a rare symptom of vaginitis, more usually associated with problems in the cervix or uterus. Bleeding between periods could be caused by the excessive irritation of a vaginal infection, but it is not a common symptom of vaginitis. When it does occur, it is usually due to trichomonas or yeast rather than gardnerella. If you have vaginal bleeding or intercourse is painful and no other symptoms of vaginitis are present, you should see your doctor immediately.

What should I do if I have any of these symptoms? Can I do anything before I see a doctor?

You must see your doctor if you have any of these symptoms. She is the only one who can diagnose the problem and give you appropriate treatment. Avoiding sexual intimacy and intercourse is a good idea so you don't transmit any infection you may have to your partner. While waiting to see your doctor, don't scratch! Applying cold, wet towels to your vulva may provide temporary relief.

What will my doctor do?

Your doctor will first take your history—ask you about your symptoms, past STDs and other diseases you may have had, what kind of birth control you use, and your sexual practices.

The gynecological examination follows, during which you will lie on your back with bent legs resting in stirrups (small metal heel supports) that spread open the knees and allow the doctor to examine the vulva to look for redness and irritation. The doctor will do a thorough pelvic exam by examining you with a gloved finger to rule out problems in the genital tract like pelvic inflammatory disease. She will place her finger deep in your vagina against your cervix, while pushing down on the lower abdomen with the other hand to detect any tenderness or enlargement of the uterus or ovaries. After this, the doctor will examine the walls of the vagina and the cervix with a speculum. The entire exam only takes a few minutes.

The diagnosis of which kind of vaginitis you have is made by taking a sample of the fluid with a cotton swab and examining it on a slide under the microscope in the office. The doctor may already have a good idea of what you have by the appearance of the discharge on the vaginal walls and on the speculum after it is removed. The yeast discharge is thick and pasty, clinging to the vaginal walls; trichomonas and gardnerella discharges are loose and very liquid.

If a diagnosis can't be made by the telltale appearance of the infectious organism under the microscope, a culture will be sent to be grown in a lab, then tested again and diagnosed. A culture should always be done in cases of vaginitis that are recurrent or have been resistant to previous treatment. Another test that can be done in the doctor's office is checking the pH of the discharge—a low, or acidic, pH is typical of yeast infections, while a high, or alkaline, pH is common for gardnerella and trichomonas. Your doctor may also add potassium hydroxide to a sample of the discharge to see if the telltale fishy odor of gardnerella can be detected.

Sometimes a routine Pap test will show trichomonas organisms even though the woman has no symptoms; this is not uncommon. All cases of both gardnerella and trichomonas should be treated even if there are no symptoms.

Your doctor may want to start treatment immediately, even before the results of the culture are known, then later adjust the treatment as needed.

How is vaginitis treated?

Gardnerella and trichomonas are treated with *metronidazole* (brand name, *Flagyl*), a prescription antibiotic that kills the trichomonas organism and the bacteria that contribute to the gardnerella infection. Metronidazole can be given as a one-day treatment: one gram by mouth morning and night. It can also be given as 250 milligrams orally three times a day over seven to ten days. Most people have no side effects, but some experience a metallic taste in the mouth, nausea, vomiting, diarrhea, or abdominal cramps. If you are allergic, you may develop a rash or hives. If you develop any of these symptoms, call your doctor.

Before metronidazole is prescribed your doctor will want to make sure you're not pregnant, and that a culture shows a definite diagnosis of trichomonas or gardnerella. You cannot take metronidazole when pregnant or breast-feeding because of possible effects on your unborn child or baby. You cannot drink alcohol while taking this drug since it prevents your body from processing the alcohol, causing nausea and vomiting. Pregnant women may be prescribed *clotrimazole (Gynelotrimin)* instead.

Metronidazole can also cause your body to produce fewer infection-fighting cells—the white blood cells. Most doctors will do a blood test, called the CBC (complete blood count), before and after treatment to monitor the white blood cell count. If you require a second course of the drug, you should definitely have a blood test.

Ampicillin, a prescription antibiotic, is sometimes chosen over metronidazole for treating gardnerella because, unlike the former, ampicillin kills the gardnerella bacteria directly instead of attacking the bacteria with which it interacts. Ampicillin only rarely has unpleasant side effects (diarrhea and mild stomach upset) and can be taken by pregnant women. The usual dose is 500 milligrams taken orally four times a day for a week. If you are allergic to penicillin, you cannot take this drug.

Yeast infections are treated with a variety of anti-fungal medications.

Miconazole (Monistat) suppositories (solid sticks of medicine that dissolve due to the moisture and heat of the vagina) are given as one 100 mg dose taken for a week or one 200 mg dose taken for three days. This drug may not be used by pregnant women because it may cause birth defects.

Clotrimazole (Mycelex or *Gynelotrimin)* is inserted into the vagina as a cream with an applicator or as a vaginal tablet. One 500-milligram cream application may give a total cure. Or it may be prescribed in lower doses: 100 mg each day for seven days or 200 mg for three days.

Butoconazole (Fem-stat) is the newest treatment alternative for yeast infection: 100 mg given orally for three days. Its effectiveness is similar to that of clotrimazole and miconazole.

Nystatin (Mycostatin), once the most common treatment, is prescribed as a suppository to be placed in the vagina twice a day (morning and evening) for one or two weeks. It can be taken in capsule, by mouth, too—either 100 mg a day for seven days or 200 mg a day for three days.

Terconazole (Terazol), available in cream or suppository form, is the newest treatment for yeast infection. Whether this new drug is more effective than the others has yet to be determined.

Side effects from all of these antifungal medications are rare, with the most common being a rash or irritation on and around the vulva that disappears when you stop using the drug. However, many are not safe during pregnancy; ask your doctor. These drugs can also weaken the latex of condoms and diaphragms and should be avoided with those products.

Note: All these drugs must be kept refrigerated to be effective. In addition, suppositories, creams, and vaginal tablets dissolve in the vagina due to body heat and moisture. They are best used when you can lie down for several hours, since they stay inside you longer that way. That's why they are most often prescribed for use at night. They can stain, so you should wear a sanitary napkin or panty liner to protect your clothes.

Gentian violet, a purple dye that prevents yeast growth, may be used instead of the antifungal antibiotics above. Painted on the vagina and vulva twice a week for several weeks by the doctor, or used by the patient in tampon form (Genapax) inserted into the vagina for four hours twice daily for twelve days, this treatment is particularly effective for recurrent yeast infections, especially those that have proved resistant to antifungal drugs. It is, however, messy and can stain clothes like suppositories and creams.

There are a variety of home remedies used by women with yeast infections. None of these self-treatments has been proven effective in scientific studies.

Some women may get temporary relief of itchiness by inserting plain yogurt into the vagina or by eating yogurt. Some doctors also recommend taking acidophilus tablets by mouth. This treatment is supposed to help the body restore the native lactobacilli that help protect the vagina against infection. Some commercial over-the-counter anti-yeast preparations contain a three percent solution of potassium sorbate, a chemical used as a food preservative. These preparations may give you some relief, though you should check with your doctor first. None of these treatments alone can completely cure vaginitis.

If I have a vaginal discharge but no other symptoms of vaginitis, what could it be?

Like skin cells, which constantly flake off from the surface to be replaced by new skin cells underneath, the **epithelial cells** on the surface of the lining of the vagina are shed constantly, but particularly so during and after the estrogen buildup (the first fourteen or so days, counting day one as the first day of your period) of the menstrual cycle. Some women shed at a higher rate than others, and they may notice what is called **physiologic leukorrhea,** a persistent whitish (from the shedding cells) discharge that can be heavy or light but is normal and not an infection. This shedding, as well as mucus secretion by the cervix, can be in response to emotional stresses like anger, anxiety, or grief or can be caused by other factors like pregnancy, obesity, sexual arousal, and even as a result of taking the birth control pill. Some women have a heavier normal discharge than others.

Many women do mistake a normal, physiologic discharge for infection, but if such a discharge is persistent or you have doubts, see your doctor. Though the condition is harmless, the symptoms—stickiness or constant wetness—can be bothersome. Douching (at your doctor's direction) with a salt-and-water or mild vinegar-and-water solution can temporarily diminish the flow. Most physiologic discharges come and go with the menstrual cycle or specific stressful periods, disappearing and coming back by themselves. Remember, though, that if you mistake a normal discharge for infection and treat yourself with old medication, you could end up with a real infection.

How can I tell if a man is infected with any of these vaginitis-causing diseases?

Because gardnerella and trichomonas are strictly sexually transmitted, it is likely that if you are infected, so is your partner. In men, these infections grow in the urethra (the tube in the penis through which urine passes from the bladder) and in the prostate gland. Male symptoms include burning during urination, a feeling that he has to urinate urgently, and wanting to urinate frequently. Many infected men, however, never have any symptoms. Thus, if you have been diagnosed with either infection, your partner needs to be treated, too.

Men rarely get yeast infections of the penis. Even if a man's partner has a severe yeast infection, the slight burning on urination or redness at the tip of the penis usually disappears by itself. Uncircumcised men can develop a whitish patch of yeast that grows underneath the foreskin at the indentation between the head and shaft of the penis, a constant source of infection for their partners if untreated. Women who get recurrent yeast infections despite treatment should ask their lovers to get checked and treated even if they don't have symptoms.

If my partner doesn't have symptoms, does he still need to be treated?

With trichomonas, the answer is yes. Avoid sexual contact until he has been treated, or he may unknowingly reinfect you, something you both want to avoid. The treatment of male partners with gardnerella is not as clear-cut. I always treat them or see that they get treatment because clinical studies have shown that male partners of women with gardnerella are often carriers, though they may have no symptoms. With yeast infections, if you have had a recurrent problem and if your partner is uncircumcised, it is wise to ask your partner to be checked to ensure that he is not the source. Otherwise, if he has no symptoms, he probably doesn't need to get treatment.

How can I avoid sexually transmitted vaginitis?

Restricting your sexual partners or having only one partner at a time decreases your chance of exposure to any STD. Using a condom, which acts to block exposure, helps, too, particularly against trichomonas and gardnerella infection. A diaphragm used with contraceptive foam also offers some protection, since it forms a barrier against the breakthrough of infectious organisms.

Keep your vulva clean and dry, since a wet vulva invites infection. You should wash your vulva at least once a day with mild soap and water; always wash after sex, and ask your partner to wash, too. After a bowel movement, wipe front to back, away from the vagina. Wearing cotton underwear and avoiding tight-fitting pantyhose or jeans allows the vagina to air, preventing excessive moisture and heat, both of which promote bacterial growth. Don't sit around in a wat bathing suit, and finally, if you are being treated for a sexually transmitted vaginal infection, don't have sex until the treatment is complete.

Special Risks and Considerations

Since vaginitis is so common, many women make the mistake of believing that they can treat it themselves, either with medication left over from previous episodes or with drugs borrowed from a friend who has also had it. Vaginitis is a condition caused, as we have seen, by different things, and the treatment must match the cause. Treating a trichomonas vaginitis with medication for yeast infections not only doesn't work but may also aggravate the condition. Gardnerella and trichomonas usually recur if the infection is resistant to the medication prescribed, if a partner doesn't get treated and so passes it on again, or if the directions for taking the prescription aren't followed. It is important to follow your doctor's instructions to the letter, get your partner treated, and otherwise minimize your risks of being reexposed.

Gardnerella Infections and Other STDs

Women with gardnerella infections are more likely to have other STDs, though gardnerella does not cause these other diseases. Pelvic inflammatory disease (PID), which is often the result of gonorrhea, chlamydia, or mycoplasma (all common STDs found more often in women with gardnerella), may occur more often in women with gardnerella. This means that if you do have gardnerella, you need to make sure you're otherwise healthy. Similarly, women who use IUDs have more gardnerella and PID than women who use other kinds of birth control. We know that gardnerella may also move up into the uterus and tubes, though whether it actually causes problems there isn't clear. It may make it easier for other infections to take hold and cause PID.

Persistent Yeast-related Vaginitis

Though we don't know why, some women have yeast infections over and over again, and the normally prescribed antifungal drugs do not cure them. Yeast can normally be present in the body—in the mouth, intestines, and vagina. Many doctors believe that yeast in the feces contaminates the nearby vagina. Also, some women's vaginal cells are particularly susceptible to yeast infections. One preventive measure for women with recurrent yeast infections is to take antifungal drugs when their doctors have prescribed antibiotics for other conditions, since antibiotics often kill the other healthy vaginal organisms that keep yeast in check. In the case of a serious and prolonged recurrence, your doctor may use the powerful antifungal *Ketoconazole*, taken by mouth, which wipes out the yeast throughout the body. As with most powerful drugs, Ketoconazole cannot be taken during pregnancy. It can also cause liver damage, and your doctor will want to monitor your liver functioning by drawing blood periodically while you take it.

Very rarely, a woman can develop an allergy to the yeast in an infection, resulting in a blotchy, red, itchy rash on the vulva that can spread to the upper thighs and anal area. The rash may ooze fluid, which forms a crust. This is treated with an antifungal cream and anti-inflammatory skin medication.

Yeast Infection and Douching

Many so-called feminine hygiene products can be harmful. Deodorants and douches are cosmetics with no medicinal value; they contain chemicals that can irritate and disturb the vagina. Douches, for instance, can alter the acidity of the vagina, creating a good environment for infection to grow—and cause vaginitis. Avoid douching unless your doctor recommends it. Spermicidal agents in contraceptive foams and jellies can also upset the balance of the vagina and help infection occur. A woman who gets vaginitis several times from a contraceptive substance should consider changing to another method.

Further Causes of Vaginitis

A puzzling problem noticed by some women is **post-sex vaginitis,** in which itching and other symptoms are experienced for a few hours after sex and then spontaneously disappear. Doctors think some women may be allergic to their partners' semen, or that the alkalinity of that semen may help offensive bacteria to grow in the vagina until the normal balance is restored by the body's natural processes. Only when other causes have been ruled out is this diagnosis possible, however. Vaginitis of this kind can be treated with a mild vinegar douche after sex, but only if your doctor recommends it.

Menopause, when the body's production of the hormone estrogen declines, can also contribute to vaginitis, since without estrogen the vagina loses its acidity, and the lining becomes thin and less resistant to infection. Estrogen replacement therapy, given only under a doctor's supervision, can provide relief from this and other menopause-related symptoms.

If You Have Vaginitis . . .
- see your doctor.
- avoid sexual contact, as you may have a sexually transmitted condition.
- try not to scratch; instead apply cool, moist towels to the vulva for relief.

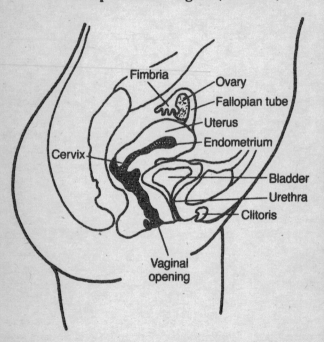

FIGURE 2:
**Anatomy of the Urinary Tract
and Reproductive Organs (side view)**

CHAPTER FOUR

Urinary Tract and Anal Infections

URINARY TRACT INFECTION (UTI)

Anatomy of the Urinary Tract

Your two kidneys, which lie on either side of your backbone under your ribs and above your waist, remove toxic (poisonous) substances and other harmful waste from the body in the form of urine. The two ureters are long tubes that carry the urine from each kidney to the bladder and are connected to it, one on either side. The bladder itself is round and smooth and, like a balloon, it expands when it fills with urine. When your bladder is full you can feel it by pressing on the abdomen, below your stomach, right above the line of your pubic hair. The urethra is the short (about one to two inches in women), straight tube that carries urine from the bladder out of the body through the small urethral opening beneath the clitoris at the top of the vulva and above the vaginal opening.

Women and UTI

Like vaginitis, **urinary tract infection (UTI)** is very common in women. Most frequently it takes the form of a **bladder infection,** or **cystitis;** but since the parts of the urinary tract are all connected, one infection can easily spread from the urethra (causing **urethritis**) to the bladder (causing **cystitis**), and from there to the kidneys (causing **pyelonephritis**). Though most UTIs are easily treated and not life-threatening, kidney infections can be very serious and can lead to widespread infection throughout the body, and possibly death in the long term if untreated.

All types of urinary infections are more common in women than men because the urethra, where the infection enters the body, is so short and so straight in women, providing an easy path for bacteria (especially from the anus and vulva) to follow.

Most UTIs are not sexually transmitted but occur when bacteria normally present in the anus and vulva come into contact with the urethra. Urethritis and cystitis in women often follow vigorous vaginal intercourse. This is not a disease transmitted by the man, but rather an irritation caused by the penis rubbing against the woman's urethra creating the conditions favorable for cystitis and urethritis to occur. It is also during intercourse that the bacteria from the vulva and anus that are directly responsible for the infection can invade the urethra.

While most UTIs are not sexually transmitted, some STDs—for example, chlamydia, mycoplasma, gonorrhea, and trichomonas (all of which are discussed in detail in other chapters)—can thrive in the urethra of men and in the urethra and vagina of women. Whether a UTI is caused by an STD or some other organism, the symptoms are similar.

Cystitis

Bladder infection, or **cystitis,** is most often caused by bacteria from the vulva, vagina, or anus gaining access to the urethra and migrating from there to the bladder. Vigorous sexual intercourse, especially for a woman who has sex infrequently, can be a factor because of the irritation of the urethra. People who, while hospitalized, have urinary catheters (the tubes inserted into the urethra to drain urine) are also more likely to develop an infection.

Most cases of cystitis are not caused by STDs. Most commonly, cystitis is caused by Escherichia coli (ninety percent of all cases) or other bacteria found in the feces like Proteus or Klebsiella. Some of the symptoms of cystitis are:

- burning pain on urination, from mild to very painful
- feeling like your bladder is full and you have to urinate urgently
- wanting to urinate often, but producing only a little urine

- getting up several times at night to urinate
- cloudy or bloody urine (which looks red or pink)
- foul-smelling urine
- feeling of pressure or pain in the bladder
- mild fever of one or two degrees

If you have any of these symptoms, you should make an appointment to see your doctor immediately. If you have had a previous UTI treated earlier by your doctor, she might renew an old prescription and tell you to begin taking it before your appointment. You should not take medicine left over from earlier UTIs without an okay from your doctor because medicine, like bread or milk, isn't good forever, and because it may not have been prescribed for the same condition. Drinking a lot of water or other fluids can help flush out the bladder and may give you some relief from the symptoms. Orange and cranberry juice, because they are so acidic, also help to destroy the bacteria in the urine.

When you see your doctor she will first examine your abdomen, looking for tenderness in the area of the bladder, then she will check the pelvis and vagina for any evidence of a vaginal or cervical infection that may also be infecting the urethra and bladder. She will ask for a urine specimen, giving you a small cloth soaked in antiseptic that you will use to cleanse the vulva before urinating. This makes sure the specimen is not con- taminated with all the normal vaginal and vulvar bacte- ria and is called a "clean catch" specimen.

Your doctor will examine the urine under the mi- croscope and also perform a urinalysis. Urinalysis is a general test that looks for sugar, blood protein, and any evidence of infection. It is also used to detect kidney problems. It tells if there is an infection; then subsequent tests can identify the particular organism. On the urinalysis, the doctor will look for large numbers of white blood cells, which signals infection. The urine culture and sensitivity tests performed by the lab will tell which organism is responsible for the infection by showing which common bacterium grows from the specimen. These tests do not, however, help identify STDs, but are excellent at determining which common bacterium is responsible for the infection. The lab will also determine which antibiotic is most effective against this particular bacterium (this is the sensitivity part of the test which takes about a day longer). Sometimes, if you've already begun taking medication or if the bacterium is present in very small numbers, the urinalysis and the urine culture will not show accurate results. If your urine culture is negative, the doctor might then look for a high number of red blood cells or excessive protein in your urine, which may indicate another problem like a kidney stone or other kidney problem.

The treatment of UTI is almost always with antibiotics, though which one is prescribed and for how long depends on your doctor and your particular case. In addition, treating cystitis caused by an STD means treating the underlying STD. (See the Table of Contents to find which diseases are covered in each chapter for specific treatments discussed in detail.) In general, a woman who develops non–STD-caused cystitis for the first time and is not pregnant could be treated with one megadose by mouth of any of the following anti-biotics: *amoxicillin, ampicillin, trimethoprim-sul-famethoxazole (Bactrim Septra)*, or *sulfisoxizole (Gantrisin)*. Pregnant women should avoid taking any drug in the sulfa or tetracycline family.

Sometimes the cure is not complete with one dose, and a more traditional, five- to ten-day course of treatment with the same medication is prescribed. This longer course is used if a woman is pregnant, has had UTIs in the past, or has a resistant UTI (one that the previously prescribed medicine doesn't cure). Since antibiotics can encourage later yeast infection, most doctors try to prescribe antibiotics for as short a time as possible.

There are many other antibiotics available. Your doctor's choice depends on her familiarity and experience with them, as well as such special considerations as penicillin allergy and side effects.

Urethritis

Urethritis (infection of the urethra), of all urinary infections, is the one most likely to be caused by a sexually transmitted disease. Women with cystitis often have urethritis, too, because the same infection moves from urethra to bladder. Sexually transmitted urethritis can be caused by chlamydia, mycoplasma, gonorrhea, trichomonas, and sometimes herpes (all covered in detail in other chapters). But STDs usually stay in the urethra and do not invade the bladder. The same organisms that cause vaginitis, especially yeast, can also cause urethritis because these organisms irritate the delicate tissues of the vulva, of which the urethral opening is a part.

Some of the symptoms of urethritis are the same as cystitis:

- mild to severe burning pain when you urinate
- having to urinate frequently and often
- cloudy or blood-tinged (pink) urine
- a small amount of opaque, whitish discharge from the urethral opening that may be difficult to see

Unlike cystitis, fever is uncommon, as is bladder pain or feeling of fullness or pressure in the bladder. Also absent in urethritis is the tenderness in the flanks that may indicate kidney infection. If the urethritis is STD-caused, you might have other symptoms of that disease, like the discharge of cervicitis in chlamydia and gonorrhea. Most women who do have urethritis caused by an STD will have evidence of infection in the cervix and pelvis as well.

If you have any of these symptoms, you should make an appointment to see your doctor as soon as you can. The doctor will first do a pelvic exam, checking for evidence of irritation or infection and "milking" your urethra (massaging it in an outward direction) to see if there is any discharge. She will also examine your cervix, uterus, and tubes and take a culture from your urethra and your cervix if she suspects an STD. The culture will be sent to a lab to be tested for the presence of gonorrhea, chlamydia, or any other STD or common bacteria. The doctor may also prepare a sample of vaginal fluid to test for trichomonas or stain a sample to look for chlamydia or gonorrhea.

The doctor will also ask for a urine sample to send for lab analysis. **Urinalysis** shows in general whether bacteria are present in the urine and the number of white blood cells present. Urinalysis can help distinguish cystitis from urethritis caused by an STD. Bacteria and the white blood cells that attack them are both present in large numbers in the urine of someone who has cystitis. Someone who has urethritis caused by an STD (which it usually is) has very few white blood cells and minimal bacteria in their urine.

Though urinalysis is a general test, it does reveal the signs of various kinds of disease. By measuring sugar and protein levels and whether there are crystals or blood in the urine, it can detect diabetes and declining kidney function. Large numbers of white blood cells or the presence of many bacteria point to possible bladder or kidney infection.

A further test, the urine culture, shows which bacteria are present in the urine by placing urine samples in a medium in which bacteria, if present, will grow in sufficient numbers to reveal the specific organism. Most doctors will use a urinalysis as the first step to help determine if an STD or a common bacteria UTI is the culprit. This is because most STDs won't show up on a routine urine culture. STDs show up on special cultures taken from the urethra so that a specific urethral culture must be taken to detect gonorrhea, mycoplasma, chlamydia, and other STDs.

Urethral cultures are done on fluid samples taken from the urethra. In men, the only way to determine what is causing urethritis is to take such a specimen, which is done by inserting a narrow-tipped swab into the urethra. This is very painful. Women more often have evidence of cervical infection at the same time, so a sample is taken from there for cervical cultures. A woman who has persistent UTIs and in whom a urinalysis only shows a few white blood cells may need a urethral culture to diagnose an STD, especially if there is no sign of infection in the cervix.

Unless your doctor finds evidence of a genital tract infection during a pelvic exam and can confirm this using a microscope in the office, you will have to wait until the tests come back, usually about a day, for treatment to begin. If urinating is painful, your doctor might begin to treat you with an antibiotic and then change the prescription once lab results are in.

As in cystitis, treating urethritis means dealing with the underlying organism causing the infection. All STD-caused urethritis is treated with antibiotics, and complete descriptions can be found in the chapters that deal with each disease. For example, the treatment of trichomonas, which is a major cause of vaginitis, is usually an antiprotozoal drug called *Flagyl*, and a complete discussion of its use can be found in the section on vaginitis. When urethritis is caused by an STD, it is necessary for both partners to be treated and not to have sexual contact until the disease has been cured.

Treating STD-caused urethritis is not complicated and usually involves taking an antibiotic, such as *doxycycline*, by mouth every day for a week. Depending on the specific bacteria, however, your doctor will treat you with any one of a variety of antibiotics. Sometimes the specific, underlying bacteria is never identified, and your doctor may treat you with a broad-spectrum (effective against a variety of bacteria) antibiotic or try a series of antibiotics until one works.

Urinary Tract Infections in Men

In men, the urethra, which runs from the bladder through the penis, is the only path for infectious organisms to enter and infect the reproductive tract. Common bacterial UTIs are *not* common in young men. If a man has symptoms of discharge, burning on urination, urinary urgency, or urinary frequency, he probably has an STD.

The discharge, perhaps only a few drops of fluid, is yellowish and creamy when gonorrhea is the infecting organism, and clearer and more watery for chlamydia and other diseases. If your partner has the painful urination and discharge (he may have to massage his urethra from base to tip of the penis to see it), have him see a doctor immediately. You should be checked, too.

Urethritis in men is similar to cervicitis in women in that urethritis is the most frequent symptom of the most common STDs like gonorrhea, chlamydia, and mycoplasma for men as cervicitis is for women with these infections. See the sections on these specific STDs for a more detailed discussion.

Recurrent UTI

For some women, bladder infections can recur even if properly treated, and those that recur are also more likely to be resistant to antibiotics. In cases where a woman has several infections in one year, her doctor may prescribe "suppression" treatment with antibiotics, which involves taking smaller doses for longer periods of time. A small dose of *Septra* or *nitrofurantoin* or some other antibiotic, for example, would be prescribed to be taken every day or every other day for several months to years (with periodic urine evaluations to check that the drug is working) to avoid any possibility of recurrence.

If you have a recurrent UTI, your doctor may prescribe an antibiotic and tell you to treat yourself at the first sign of infection. Women who develop symptoms after intercourse can take an antibiotic before sex and avoid the flare-up.

Infection without Symptoms: Asymptomatic UTI

Sometimes a doctor will find evidence of infection in the results of a routine urinalysis (many white blood cells and the presence of bacteria) even though you have no symptoms. This is especially common in pregnant women, who have a much higher incidence of cystitis (bladder infection) and pyelonephritis (kidney infection), although no one knows exactly why. Asymptomatic infections should be treated just as seriously as those with symptoms because, untreated, they can recur with all the symptoms and lead to cystitis and pyelonephritis. Pregnant women should be alert for any sign of UTI and have their urine checked as their doctor directs. If you are pregnant and have either a recurring or new UTI, your doctor will not prescribe one-shot megadose treatment but will probably want to treat you with smaller doses for at least a week.

Antibiotics in the *sulfa* and *tetracycline* families should not be taken during pregnancy, so your doctor will probably choose one from another group.

Preventing Urinary Infections

You can prevent urinary tract infections by following these guidelines:

- Use a condom or other barrier contraceptive.
- Use lubrication like K-Y Jelly for intercourse, to avoid irritation of your urethra if your own vaginal lubrication is not adequate.
- Intercourse with your partner on top of you causes the most friction against the urethra, so you may want to try another position. Having intercourse side by side or with you on top is better when friction is a problem. Anal sex is *not* a good idea, since anal bacteria on his penis can later contaminate your vagina and urethra and transmit other STDs.
- Try to urinate within half an hour after intercourse to flush out the bladder and urethra. Drinking some liquids beforehand will help you to do this.
- If your vagina feels sore or irritated during intercourse, stop.
- Shower and wash carefully after intercourse but avoid washing your vulva with a lot of soap. Deodorant soaps can be very irritating to the vulva and urethra. Vaginal deodorant sprays and deodorant sanitary pads can also irritate the urethra.
- After going to the bathroom, wipe front to back so that fecal matter will not be close to your vulva.

- Urinate when you feel you have to, since a full bladder is a good place for bacteria to grow.
- Make sure your jeans, pantyhose, and undergarments are not too tight.
- If you have frequent urinary infections, it is a good idea to cut down on coffee, tea, cola soft drinks, and alcoholic beverages.

Women who use a diaphragm are three times more likely to get cystitis. This is because the rim of the diaphragm puts pressure against the urethra where it enters the bladder. This can stop the bladder from emptying completely and make it more susceptible to any bacteria that might be present in the urine. When using a diaphragm you should urinate both before and after intercourse. You may want to be fitted for a smaller diaphragm if possible, since the smaller it is the less pressure it puts on the urethra. Contraceptive jellies and foams used alone or with a diaphragm can also irritate the urethra. If UTIs become a recurrent problem, talk to your doctor about changing your birth control method. This is important because cystitis can lead to kidney infection and increase the chance of an infection becoming resistant to antibiotics.

INFECTIONS OF THE ANUS AND RECTUM

The anus is the round, muscle-rimmed opening surrounded by the buttocks through which fecal matter is eliminated from the body. The anus is the end point of the rectum, which is a short tube that leads to the intestinal system. The anus and rectum are lined with a very thin, extremely delicate membrane that receives a large blood supply. This membrane is easily torn or irritated by the insertion of a penis, sex tool, or any other foreign object, creating an easy entry for infection.

Infections of the anus and rectum—which are called **proctitis**—occur when bacteria penetrate the rectal tissue. Though bacteria are present normally in the anus in fecal waste, the tissue of the anal membrane prevents their entering the body. It is usually only when trauma occurs—the small tears and abrasions caused by the penis during anal intercourse, for example—that bacteria enter at the vulnerable site to cause infection. If you do not practice anal intercourse or insert sex tools like vibrators into the anus, you have practically no risk of getting anal or rectal infections. If you do have anal sex, you can get chlamydia, gonorrhea, herpes, syphilis, or warts from having anal intercourse with an infected man. Having vigorous anal sex or using sex tools anally irritates the rectum and anus, making it easier not only for STDs but also for the bacteria normally present there to cause infection.

The symptoms of proctitis are:

- painful defecation and soreness of the anal area
- puslike or blood-tinged discharge from the anus
- bleeding from the anus, which you may notice as streaks of blood on toilet paper after wiping or as stains on your underwear
- with herpes: a numbness or tingling followed by very painful blisters and sores
- with syphilis: the painless chancre (sore)

- with anal warts: painless fleshy growths in and around the anus, often internal and invisible

If you have any of these symptoms, even if you don't practice anal intercourse, see your doctor immediately. One of the most common problems affecting the anus—hemorrhoids—shares some of the symptoms of proctitis. Hemorrhoids resemble pieces of flesh that rim the anus. But hemorrhoids are actually the result of dilated and enlarged veins, and they can itch, burn, and bleed and make defecating painful. Hemorrhoids are not an STD and are quite common. They require treatment only if the pain and itching are constant or if the bleeding is severe.

When you go to the doctor, she will examine your buttocks and anus with a gloved finger, looking for redness, discharge, and the presence of any sores like those that occur in herpes and syphilis. If there is a discharge, she will take a sample to be analyzed in the lab. She will insert a gloved finger into the anus and feel the walls of the rectum looking for tender spots and internal sores. She may also want to use an **anoscope,** a long, narrow tube with lenses at both ends that allows the doctor to examine the rectal walls as if through a telescope. This is a painful procedure, and your doctor will probably want to give you a sedative before performing it.

Though proctitis is common among homosexual men, it is rare even in women who do have anal sex. Other, non–STD-caused diseases that can infect the bowel are protozoal parasites like the amoeba and giardia and bacterial organisms like shigella and salmonella. But these infections almost never occur in a heterosexual woman unless her partner is a gay or bisexual man. Symptoms of these diseases include diarrhea, foul-smelling stools, a bloated feeling in the abdomen, and unexplained weight loss. Among homosexual men these infections are epidemic, often occurring together in what doctors call "gay bowel syndrome."

If you do have proctitis, temporary relief can be provided by sitz baths using drugstore preparations and by avoiding long periods sitting down. Treatment is specific to the organism that underlies the infection and mostly involves taking antibiotics. See the specific diseases discussed in other chapters for specific treatment information.

The best way to avoid or prevent anal infections is not to have anal sex.

PART
III

Gonorrhea, Chlamydia, Mycoplasma, and Pelvic Inflammatory Disease

Gonorrhea, chlamydia, and mycoplasma are potentially dangerous STDs like syphilis and herpes that may, if untreated, lead to the more complex disease syndrome of the pelvis known as **pelvic inflammatory disease (PID)**. PID is a ravaging disease that infects, inflames, and later scars the uterus, tubes, and ovaries. Doctors call gonorrhea, chlamydia, and mycoplasma "ascending" diseases because these infections settle in the cervix and may later "ascend" or rise up to the uterine lining (the endometrium) and from there to the fallopian tubes and even the ovaries.

The effects of these ascending diseases can be moderate, as in cervicitis, but are often severe, causing, for example, infection of the endometrium and fallopian tubes, which can spread throughout the whole pelvis. This is PID. In PID the infection is severe enough to cause inflammation of all the upper reproductive organs, and the resulting scarring of the fallopian tubes and uterus can cause tubal pregnancies, miscarriages, or infertility long after the initial infection.

To make it easier to distinguish between the syndromes and the diseases that cause them, the diseases are presented first, in question-and-answer format, so that symptoms, prevention, and other important information will be clear in your mind. The second chapter of Part Three covers the more complex syndromes that result from these diseases, explaining what they are, how they occur, and what to do if you have them.

Anatomy of the Cervix and Upper Pelvic Organs

The vagina, smooth-walled and lined with tough epithelial cells, is the passage between the outside world and the uterus. The external genitals or vulva (labia, urethral opening, clitoris, etc.) are at one end, with the cervix at the other, where it forms the base of the uterus above, connecting it to the vagina. The cervix acts as a divider between the upper genital tract (the reproductive organs—uterus, fallopian tubes, and ovaries) and the lower genital tract (the vagina and the

FIGURE 3:
Anatomy of the Reproductive Organs
(side view)

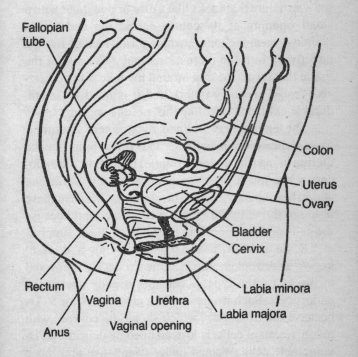

rest of the vulva). You can feel your cervix if you squat down and insert your index or middle finger deep into your vagina. The cervix will feel rubbery, but also firm and smooth.

Looking through your vagina at the cervix (which is how your doctor sees it when she inserts the speculum to push back the muscular vaginal walls), you will see a structure that looks like a disc or doughnut with a small opening at its center called the **endocervix** ("endo-" meaning inner), which forms a canal leading directly up into the uterus, or womb. The rest of the tissue that forms the disc around the hole is the **exocervix** ("exo-" meaning outer), and it is lined by tough, durable epithelial cells like those of the vagina.

The endocervix is lined by thinner, smoother, more delicate epithelial cells like those found in the uterine lining (the endometrium). The cells of the endocervix are much more open to attack by STDs like gonorrhea, chlamydia, and mycoplasma because these diseases thrive in the upper genital tract and because the cells of the endocervix have a large blood supply.

Some women have a condition (not a disease) known as **ectropion,** in which the exocervix is covered in places by the type of cell that usually covers the endocervix. Such women are at a greater risk for STDs because the exocervix, which should be covered with tough, resistant cells, is instead lined by delicate, STD-vulnerable cells. Women under twenty-five and those who use birth control pills are more likely to have ectropion, which makes them in turn more likely to get cervicitis and, thus, upper genital tract STDs (though ectropion is not directly responsible). Ectropion is not a permanent condition, and most women grow out of it.

The endocervix serves as the entry for sperm and as an exit for menstrual fluid and a passage for the baby during birth. Leading directly into the uterus, it also serves as the uterus's mouth or neck, supporting the uterus by forming a barrel-shaped stand on which the uterus sits.

The uterus is shaped like an upside-down pear, with a wide dome at its top that gradually tapers down to the cervix, its narrowest part. The innermost layer of tissue of the uterus is the **endometrium,** a velvety smooth lining of delicate cells like those of the endo-cervix. The cells of the uterine lining are so smooth and richly fed by the bloodstream because the uterus is where the fertilized egg, which needs the nutrients provided by the blood to grow, will attach itself and develop into a fetus. The next layer going outward from the uterine lining is the **myometrium,** a layer of muscle about an inch thick.

The major function of the uterus is to hold and feed the fetus during pregnancy. The network of mus-cle fibers of the myometrium allows the uterus to stretch from its normal size of a pear to the size of a watermelon in late pregnancy. The rhythmic, forceful squeezing or contractions of the myometrium (labor) push the baby through the vagina out into the world during birth and expel menstrual fluid during your pe-riod.

When the uterus becomes infected from an STD, it is almost always the endometrium or lining that is affected because any organism that reaches the cervix can easily move up into the endometrium through the endocervix. The endometrium's rich blood supply and delicate cells provide the kind of environment such infections prefer and thrive in. Another good environment for an infectious organism's growth exists, of course, during menstruation. Gonorrhea, for example, is more likely to ascend from the cervix to the pelvic organs during menstruation.

The ovaries look like small, firm, flattened, hard-boiled eggs about one and a half inches wide, and they sit on either side of the top of the uterus, connected to it by the fallopian tubes. They produce eggs (ova) as well as the female sex hormones, and each contains several hundred thousand ripening eggs, though only one egg ripens to full size and is released during each month into the fallopian tubes at ovulation.

The fallopian tubes are thin, delicate, droopy pink tubes that run about five inches between the ovaries and uterus. At the uterus, each tube is about one inch thick; in the middle, about as wide as a telephone cord. At the ovary, each tube flares open and is shaped like a blooming tulip. This is called the fimbria, and this part of the tube contains millions of very thin, silklike strands of tissue whose function is to draw out and bring an egg from the ovary into the tube itself. The tubes are very smoothly lined so that the egg and the sperm that will fertilize it there have an easy passage. The sperm moves from the uterus through the tube to reach the egg, and the now-fertilized egg moves back down into the uterus, where it will attach itself. Any blockage or scarring of the tubes (and ovaries) can make this downward passage difficult or impossible, leading to long-term fertility problems.

All of the inner reproductive organs sit in the lower abdomen, the lower part of the belly below the waist. They are surrounded by loops of intestine. The bladder, which holds urine, sits in front of the uterus, right below the belly button. The whole abdomen is lined by a thin but very strong membrane, the peritoneum. When pelvic organs like the ovaries and fallopian tubes get infected from an STD, they can infect the peritoneum. The infection can reach other organs like the liver and appendix via the peritoneum, causing pain and tenderness throughout the whole adomen.

CHAPTER FIVE

Gonorrhea, Chlamydia, and Mycoplasma

GONORRHEA

What is gonorrhea?

Until recently, **gonorrhea** was the most common (and infamous) STD. There are still about two million cases of gonorrhea reported each year in the U.S., though the real number of cases is believed to be at least twice as high. Caused by the bacterium Neisseria gonorrhea, gonorrhea is a disease that lives in the moist tissues of the body—usually the cervix in women or the urethra in men—though it can also invade other parts of the body, in both sexes, if contracted in those places. Though it often goes unnoticed in women, producing no symptoms, it meanwhile causes infection in the cervix and can rise up into the uterus, fallopian tubes, and entire pelvis. Untreated, it spreads throughout the body in the bloodstream and over time can lead to serious conditions such as arthritis, endocarditis (infection of the heart), and meningitis, which can be fatal.

How do you get gonorrhea?

Gonorrhea is transmitted through intimate sexual contact with the moist tissue of an infected person, such as occurs in anal and vaginal intercourse and oral sex. Since the disease lives in moist tissue—in men the anus, throat, and urethra—any contact with these mucous membranes can lead to transmission, though vaginal intercourse is how most women get it. If a woman has oral sex with an infected man and he is the passive partner, for example, she can get gonorrhea in her mouth from swallowing his sperm or getting infectious secretions in her mouth. A woman can also get gonorrhea if she gets his semen on her hands while touching or masturbating him, then touching her vulva or her mouth, though this is not common. It is very unlikely that an infected man could transmit gonorrhea to a woman from his mouth while performing oral sex on her, or that a man could catch gonorrhea by performing oral sex on an infected woman.

What are the symptoms of gonorrhea in women?

Most women who contract gonorrhea do not notice any symptoms since gonorrhea invades the cervix rather than the vagina, producing inflammation, a condition called **muco-purulent cervicitis** ("muco-" means mucous and "purulent" means full of pus), usually about a week after infection. The infected cervix produces a creamy white discharge, but this usually passes unnoticed since it mixes with vaginal secretions, which just makes them slightly thicker. Other symptoms that can but don't always occur are a mild burning on urination and urinary frequency—feeling like you have to urinate often—both of which happen when the bacterium invades the urethra. Gonorrhea can also cause a Bartholin's gland infection, which is usually painful and therefore noticeable.

Occasionally, women with gonorrhea may feel pain during sexual intercourse or have some bleeding after sex. There may also be a dull, throbbing pain in the pelvis accompanied by fever and chills. These symptoms—the pain and fever—may mean that the infection has spread beyond the cervix to the uterus, fallopian tubes, and ovaries, which is then called pelvic inflammatory disease. Severe infection of the cervix or pelvic organs can cause dull, throbbing lower back pain as well. Though gonorrhea spreads to the upper pelvic organs in only about twenty percent of all women who have it, PID is a very serious condition that requires immediate medical attention.

What symptoms do men have? How can I tell if my partner has gonorrhea?

Eighty percent of men infected with gonorrhea will have symptoms when the infection settles into the narrow tube of the urethra. Only twenty percent of women with gonorrhea will have symptoms. From two to seven days after being infected a man will experience pain when urinating, will feel he has to urinate frequently, and may notice a yellowish-white puslike discharge from the tip of his penis that may stain underwear. The skin around the urethral opening at the tip of the penis can also become reddened and irritated. Less commonly, the infection can spread to the epididymis (the tubes in the scrotum that store sperm) and the prostate gland.

How does gonorrhea affect the throat and the anus?

In men and women, gonorrhea of the anus and rectum causes painful bowel movements, anal pain and itching, and a bloody, puslike discharge from the anus. Though this condition is more frequent in male homosexuals, heterosexual women who practice anal intercourse can also get it.

For men and women with pharyngeal gonorrhea (in the throat), swallowing is painful and their tonsils can become swollen from the infection. It occurs much more frequently in those who perform oral sex on an infected man than in those who perform oral sex on an infected woman.

If gonorrhea has no noticeable symptoms, how will my doctor diagnose it?

Most of the time, women discover they have gonorrhea only after their partners develop symptoms, or when their doctors find evidence of infection in the cervix during a routine gynecological exam. In the worst case, fertility problems may lead to the discovery that a woman has gonorrhea and the more complex syndrome, PID. If your partner has any of the symptoms, especially the discharge from the penis, you should see your doctor as soon as possible.

The doctor will first examine you with a speculum and, if she notices a reddened cervix and evidence of a puslike discharge from the center of the cervix, will take a swab of the discharge for laboratory testing for gonorrhea. Then the doctor will do a manual exam, inserting a gloved finger deep into the vagina and pressing against the cervix, then pressing down on the abdomen from the outside with the other hand to detect any inflammation or tenderness of the pelvic organs. Evidence of inflammation or pain during this procedure may mean that the uterus, fallopian tubes, or ovaries have been infected as well—all signs of the condition known as pelvic inflammatory disease, which occurs in at least one fifth of all women who have gonorrhea.

If there is evidence of muco-purulent cervicitis, the doctor will examine a sample of the fluid under the microscope. Sometimes the bacteria will show up immediately after the sample has been treated with a special stain, and your doctor will begin appropriate treatment right away. To confirm the diagnosis, or if the test was performed as a routine screen, the sample will be sent to a lab to be cultured to see if gonorrhea bacteria grow from it. This usually takes two days to a week.

How is gonorrhea treated?

Gonorrhea can be cured very quickly and dependably with antibiotics. To avoid reinfection, both partners should be treated simultaneously, and both partners should be retested after treatment to be certain the cure is total. One factor considered in gonorrhea treatment is that the disease occurs in combination with **chlamydia** (another bacterial STD discussed in the next section of this chapter) about half the time, and with **syphilis,** too, though much less frequently. For this reason, if you are being tested for gonorrhea, your doctor will probably test for chlamydia and may test for syphilis. The treatment for gonorrhea usually includes treatment for chlamydia as well, since they occur so often together.

For localized, uncomplicated gonorrhea (gonorrhea that has not spread beyond the cervix), treatment can be:

- a single dose of *amoxicillin*, six 500-milligram capsules taken by mouth at the same time, followed by two 500-milligram capsules of *probenecid*, a drug that enables the amoxicillin to stay in your system longer to kill the bacteria.

or

- a single dose of *ampicillin,* seven 500-milligram capsules taken by mouth at the same time, followed by *probenecid* as above.

or

- *penicillin* given as 2.4 million units injected in two different places, usually both buttocks, followed by *probenecid* as above.

All of the above treatments are for the gonorrhea alone and are usually followed by antibiotic treatment against chlamydia, which is:

- *tetracycline,* 500 milligrams taken by mouth four times daily for seven to ten days. *Tetracycline* does not cause side effects in most people. However, some people do suffer stomach upset or cramping. Sunbathing should be avoided since the drug can make the skin more sensitive and cause rashes. Your doctor will also tell you to avoid certain foods and products which contain calcium (milk, antacids, vitamin supplements) since these interfere with the body's ability to absorb the drug. *Tetracycline* should not be taken by pregnant women since it can cause birth defects.

or

- *doxycycline* (a drug much like tetracycline) 100–200 milligrams taken orally twice a day for a week. *Doxycycline,* a newer derivative of *tetracycline,* is more expensive but seems to cause less stomach upset. Your doctor will tell you to stay out of the sun since the drug can also cause the skin to be sensitive to exposure.

In cases where the woman is pregnant or allergic to tetracycline, *erythromycin,* 500 milligrams taken four times daily for a week, is substituted. In those allergic to penicillin (and to ampicillin and amoxicillin, which are related to it), tetracycline or doxycycline alone is given, but for ten days. This is often accompanied by an injection of the antibiotic *spectinomycin* (a two-gram dose) or *ceftriaxone* (a 250-milligram dose).

What else could it be?

Often the painful urination, increased urge to urinate, and puslike discharge from a gonorrheal infection are mistaken for symptoms of the more common cystitis or urinary tract infection. Some women may try to treat themselves with medication left over from previous bouts with these illnesses. This only postpones the visit to the doctor and allows the infection to spread.

Any infection of the urethra, STD or otherwise, causes burning on urination and urinary frequency. Most women who get urethritis from gonorrhea will usually have gonorrhea in the cervix, causing mucopurulent cervicitis. Unless you have other symptoms, only your doctor can tell, by testing your urine, the cause of the urinary symptoms.

If you have a discharge from your vagina but don't think you've been exposed to gonorrhea, it could be a vaginal infection or vaginitis. Again, it is very hard to tell the discharge of gonorrhea-caused cervicitis from that of other infections. With any unusual discharge you should see your doctor.

How can I avoid getting gonorrhea?

Practicing safe sex is the best way to avoid the disease. Condoms and diaphragms used with spermicidal foam or jelly are especially protective because the chemical in spermicide kills (some, not necessarily all of) the gonorrhea germ. Because you may not always notice the symptoms, *you should be routinely tested for gonorrhea if you have more than one sexual partner a year and do not use a barrier-type contraceptive like the diaphragm or condom.*

Special Risks and Considerations

Gonorrhea and Pregnancy

A woman infected with gonorrhea can pass it to her newborn during childbirth. The disease can infect the eyes, throat, lungs, or skin of the infant, though the routine use of silver nitrate drops in the eyes of newborns has vastly decreased infant gonococcal eye infections. Infant gonorrhea is usually not life-threatening if treated immediately.

Gonorrhea and Infertility

Gonorrhea is responsible for at least one fifth of all cases of PID, which is a major cause of infertility in women. A complete discussion of the effects of gonorrhea on fertility is provided in the section on pelvic inflammatory disease.

Penicillin-Resistant Gonorrhea

Penicillin-resistant gonorrhea used to be confined to Southeast Asia and South America, but today it is seen increasingly in the U.S., especially in New York City, Los Angeles, and parts of Florida. These cases can be treated with other antibiotic drugs like *spectinomycin, cefoxitin,* or *ceftriaxole* instead of simple penicillin. Usually the culture and sensitivity tests done on a specimen show which drugs will work. Since drug-resistant gonorrhea does exist, however, it is important to be tested after treatment no matter what drug you've been treated with to make certain the cure is effective.

If You Have Gonorrhea . . .

- see your doctor immediately to get tested and treated.
- tell your partner or anyone you've been intimate with so that he can get treatment.
- you might, when you are examined, have an abnormal Pap smear because of the cervicitis gonorrhea causes. After treatment the cervix should return to normal and the atypical changes reverse, but this is something that should be monitored by your doctor.
- and the infection has spread to your pelvic organs,

your doctor may want to do diagnostic tests after treatment to determine the damage, if any.

CHLAMYDIA

Chlamydia is a bacterial STD caused by the organism chlamydia trachomatis. It can survive only in the cells it invades and hence cannot live outside the body on the skin. It is now the most common STD in the U.S., with anywhere from three to ten million cases a year, though the true number of cases is not known since doctors aren't required to report it as they must syphilis and gonorrhea.

Doctors and other health care workers often call chlamydia "the silent epidemic" because, though millions of men and women are infected, the disease produces no symptoms for weeks to months, and sometimes for years. In women the disease follows the same course as gonorrhea. It first invades the cervix, causing muco-purulent cervicitis, then rises into the uterus and other pelvic organs. Often it is first detected only after developing into pelvic inflammatory disease, which can cause great damage to the reproductive organs and even threaten a woman's fertility. Chlamydia is responsible for at least ten percent of all cases of symptomatic or acute PID and many more cases of pelvic scarring.

How is chlamydia transmitted?

Sexual intercourse or any kind of intimacy that involves exposure of your genitals to your partner's secretions or fluids—semen or vaginal and cervical secretions—can transmit chlamydia. As with gonorrhea, vaginal intercourse is how most chlamydia is transmitted, but (also like gonorrhea) you can also get chlamydia from the vaginal secretions or semen and sperm of an infected person when these fluids touch your mucous membranes. Though there are cases of chlamydia infecting a person's eyes, it is found mostly in the genital areas of men and women.

What are the symptoms of chlamydia?

Chlamydia is often "silent"; it is less likely than gonorrhea to cause pain on urination, fever, or pelvic tenderness. And when the symptoms do occur, they are often so mild as to be unnoticeable. When the infection first establishes itself in the cervix, the first sign is muco-purulent cervicitis, in which the cervix becomes inflamed and produces a small amount of pale yellow or white puslike discharge. Because the discharge mixes with normal vaginal secretions and is often light to begin with, many women don't notice it at all.

From the cervix, chlamydia, like gonorrhea, can spread to the uterus, fallopian tubes, and ovaries, still without further symptoms. Some women may notice a slight cramping pressure or a deep aching sensation in the lower abdomen around the area of the pelvic organ or in the lower back. It is usually only when the disease is firmly established in the pelvic organs that the classic symptoms of pelvic inflammatory disease occur. These are high fever accompanied by severe pelvic pain and tenderness in the lower abdomen. Other symptoms of chlamydia's infection of the pelvic organs are painful sexual intercourse, abnormal vaginal bleeding, and bleeding after sexual intercourse, though these symptoms do not occur in all women. Finally, chlamydia can also invade the urethra and bladder, causing burning when urinating and the desire to urinate frequently. Though the symptoms are similar to gonorrhea, they are usually milder when they do occur. Acute PID, with fever, pain, and tenderness, is also less common with chlamydia than with gonorrhea.

What symptoms does chlamydia cause in men?

In men, chlamydia's symptoms, like those of gonorrhea, occur in the urethra, the thin tube that runs through the penis carrying urine from the bladder. Chlamydia in men is, in fact, called nongonococcal urethritis (NGU). Unlike women, many men do have symptoms, though these are not as striking as what they would experience with gonorrhea's symptoms. When the chlamydia infection settles there it causes painful urination and the feeling of needing to urinate frequently. Men can also have a clear or pale yellow discharge from the tip of the penis that is less thick, less opaque, and less puslike than the gonorrhea discharge. Some new evidence also indicates that chlamydia can attack sperm, rendering them infertile. Some men will never have symptoms and so may pass it on to their partners.

If chlamydia is "silent," causing no symptoms, how will I know if I have it?

As with gonorrhea, women often discover the disease only after their male partners begin to show symptoms, or when their doctors find it during a routine gynecological exam. Unfortunately, some women will discover chlamydia after they experience symptoms of the more complex syndrome, PID. Acute PID with fever and severe abdominal pain is, for chlamydia, the exception and not the rule. Though many women will have no symptoms at all and others symptoms so mild (like abdominal cramping or tenderness) they mistake them for premenstrual pain or backache, some women do discover the infection when they have other symptoms like a burning sensation when urinating or a heavier vaginal discharge.

As chlamydia has become more common in recent years many doctors have begun testing their patients regularly for chlamydia, even if no symptoms are present. Because it is a silent epidemic and often does not have easily diagnosed symptoms, *you should be routinely tested for chlamydia if you have more than one sexual partner a year and do not use a barrier-type contraceptive like the diaphragm or condom*, both of which prevent chlamydia from reaching the cervix.

What will my doctor do to test for chlamydia?

If your doctor finds muco-purulent cervicitis or you have pelvic pain or tenderness during a gynecological examination, or even just routinely, she will want to test for chlamydia, gonorrhea, or other STDs that could be causing the symptoms.

As with gonorrhea, the quickest, easiest way for a doctor to diagnose chlamydia is by looking at a sample of the discharge under the microscope. She adds a special stain to the sample that makes the white blood cells stand out. Since these cells have "eaten" the infectious organisms, they stand out, too. This procedure can be done while you wait and can diagnose chlamydia in about three out of four cases.

The most accurate test is a culture, in which a sample of cervical fluid or, in men, of the penile discharge is placed in a specially prepared culture kit. If the disease is present, the bacteria will grow on the culture dish. The procedure is eighty percent accurate (the most accurate of all tests), takes two days, and costs about $100. It is almost always used to confirm the diagnosis made on the basis of the microscopic examination of a fluid sample described above.

The most commonly used test is **chlamydia immunofluorescence.** It is cheaper—about $35—but still pretty reliable and uses a fluid sample like the culture. The sample is stained in the lab with a substance that, under a special microscope, causes the chlamydia bacteria to glow.

There is also a blood test for chlamydia, the **enzyme immunoassay test,** which measures the number of antibodies (disease-fighting cells) in the blood that have developed in response to the disease. This will reliably show if you have ever had chlamydia but does not help the doctor determine if you have it presently, or which organs are involved and to what extent.

Chlamydia is difficult to detect because it may have no symptoms. Sometimes the test is negative when the infection has spread beyond the cervix to the uterus or fallopian tubes. The infection may have retreated from the cervix or be present in very small quantities. A culture test made from cervical secretions may then show no chlamydia even though the disease is present higher up in the pelvis. In this case, when the doctor has other reasons to suspect the uterus or fallopian tubes may be infected (like fever or pelvic tenderness and pain, or when a woman is having problems getting pregnant), she may want to take specimens for testing from those areas.

A uterine specimen—called an **endometrial biopsy**—can be taken in the doctor's office. The doctor may first give you a shot of painkiller where the sample is to be taken. Then she will pass a curette—a scraping instrument with a small spoon-shaped tip that can remove a thin strand of tissue—through the opening in the cervix into the uterine cavity. The labia are spread open first with the speculum so that the instrument won't nick or cut you as it is inserted. The curette cuts a small tissue sample from the endocervix or endometrium, the tissue that lines the uterus. The tissue is then cultured and tested. Though this procedure is performed under local anesthesia, many women will have moderate to severely painful abdominal cramps afterwards. The cramps may last for several hours and sometimes several days, but they can be lessened by taking *ibuprofen* (brand names *Advil, Motrin,* or *Nuprin*) an hour before the procedure and then later as necessary.

If a woman has an enlargement of, or mass in, her fallopian tube or ovary or is having difficulty getting pregnant, the doctor may want to do a **laparoscopy**. An exploratory laparoscopy is a procedure done in a hospital in which a lighted lens tube is inserted into a one-inch cut below the navel. If general anesthesia is not used, the doctor will anesthetize the site of the cut with an injection of local anesthesia before the incision is made. Through the tube the doctor can examine the abdomen and all the pelvic organs including the fallopian tubes for signs of STD-related infection and scarring damage and take small tissue samples. This procedure is quite common and is often used to confirm other diagnoses relating to problems like endometriosis and ovarian cysts or to make sure a tubal pregnancy has not occurred when a woman has some symptoms but is not acutely ill. Laparoscopy is also the procedure used for tubal ligation—tying the tubes for sterilization. Most women can leave the hospital the same day, but sometimes overnight hospitalization is necessary. Usually the procedure is done under general anesthesia.

How is chlamydia treated? Can it be cured?

Chlamydia, like gonorrhea, is effectively treated and cured with antibiotics. The treatment for uncomplicated chlamydia, or chlamydia cervicitis, and its male counterpart nongonococcal urethritis, is the same. Since chlamydia and gonorrhea can occur together in acute PID, most doctors treat them together. If you have only chlamydia in your cervix, your doctor may prescribe tetracycline or doxycycline by itself. Refer to the section on gonorrhea for the details of your treatment.

If it's not chlamydia, what else can it be?

Pain when urinating and urinary frequency occur when any infection—gonorrhea, chlamydia, or non-STD urethritis or cystitis, for example—settles in the urethra. If you only have these two symptoms, then you probably have a urinary tract infection, though only your doctor can tell for sure by testing your urine. Severe cramps could mean endometriosis, PID, or sometimes gonorrhea when they happen when you're not having your period. A vaginal discharge, when it occurs alone, might only be vaginitis and not a more serious STD, but again, any unusual discharge should get you to the doctor quickly. Like gonorrhea, the symptoms of chlamydia are not always obvious and easy to spot yourself. When you notice something unusual or different—cramps when you're not expecting to get your period, a discharge that smells bad, or unexplained pain—your body is trying to tell you something. See your doctor.

How can I avoid getting chlamydia?

Since men show the symptoms much more frequently than women (at least half of all men who are infected with chlamydia have symptoms), look for the signs—the reddened tip of the penis, frequent urination with pain, whitish-yellow discharge—before being intimate. Ask if he's had urethritis recently and been treated for it.

Using a condom with spermicide will help protect you from chlamydia. Women who use barrier contraceptives—condoms and diaphragms—are much less likely, when they have chlamydia, to develop PID because the contraceptive prevents the disease from passing from your partner's penis to your cervix and other pelvic organs. Limiting the number of your sexual partners reduces your risk of exposure even more.

Because chlamydia can be "silent," have a test for chlamydia as part of a routine gynecological checkup. If you already have the disease, you can get it treated quickly and effectively before it causes PID and affects your fertility.

Finally, if you are planning to become pregnant by artificial insemination, be sure the sperm bank screens for chlamydia.

Gonorrhea and chlamydia seem alike. How are they different?

Gonorrhea and chlamydia are both bacteria; both establish themselves in the cervix but can rise up to cause PID; and both can have no symptoms. Gonorrhea and chlamydia are also very similar in the symptoms they cause and the later conditions they produce—like PID—if undetected. Gonorrhea cervicitis, or nongonococcal urethritis in men, however, produces a different discharge, one that is usually thicker and more opaque and puslike. Chlamydia discharge is more watery. The major difference between the two is that gonorrhea, if it ascends the uterus to become PID, is much more likely to cause the acute syndrome of severe abdominal pain, tenderness, and fever. Chlamydia is more likely to be asymptomatic, causing a condition called "silent PID." Though gonorrhea causes acute PID condition, chlamydia-related PID is more likely to cause infertility. Also, after establishing itself in the cervix, chlamydia is about twice as likely to rise and infect the pelvic organs, although it usually does this silently.

Special Risks and Considerations

Chlamydia and Pregnancy

You can pass chlamydia to your baby in the birth canal, and it can cause eye infections and pneumonia. Chlamydia does not usually threaten the life of the newborn. Chlamydia prevents conception—via PID scarring—rather than complicating pregnancy.

Chlamydia and Post-Surgical PID

Many doctors will do a chlamydia test before performing any kind of pelvic surgery because sometimes it is only after such an operation that a chlamydia infection already present there causes the acute-PID syndrome. The surgical instruments used in an abortion, dilatation and curettage, Caesarean section, endometrial biopsy, the aftermath of a miscarriage, or sometimes even in normal vaginal delivery may introduce the chlamydia further into the genital tract, "stirring things up" and activating the symptoms. The symptoms are fever, foul-smelling or bloody vaginal discharge, abdominal pain or tenderness, or tenderness during any part of a pelvic exam.

If You Have Chlamydia . . .
- see your doctor immediately.
- avoid sexual contact until after you've been treated and tested again.
- inform your sex partners and be sure they get treatment.
- and you are pregnant, get treatment immediately.

MYCOPLASMA

Mycoplasma are very small bacteria that lack cell walls, which makes them like viruses in many ways. They can cause disease in many parts of the body—infections in the middle ear and pneumonia in the lungs, for example. The mycoplasmas that cause disease in the genitals are called Mycoplasma hominis and Ureaplasma ureolyticum. Mycoplasma as an STD is much rarer than gonorrhea or chlamydia, but it is getting more common. Because it is rare, the disease has not been widely studied, and much about it is still unknown. However, each year more and more cases are being reported. Mycoplasma can be found in the reproductive tracts of many healthy, sexually active people who do not have symptoms or evidence of disease.

Like gonorrhea and chlamydia, mycoplasma causes a whole range of diseases, beginning with infection of the cervix (cervicitis) and in some cases going on to cause acute PID. Though mycoplasma is only responsible for about five percent of all cases of PID, it often occurs with chlamydia and gonorrhea, which together cause more PID than anything else.

Like gonorrhea and chlamydia, mycoplasma is transmitted by any kind of sexual intimacy where one person's genitals are exposed to the fluids or secretions of another—sperm, semen, and vaginal and cervical secretions. Mycoplasma, once transmitted, follows the same course as chlamydia, with the same symptoms (see previous section for complete information). It first settles in the cervix and, if untreated, ascends to the endometrium and tubes to cause PID. Its effects are similar, too—pelvic scarring that, though not as severe as chlamydia, is responsible for infertility and tubal pregnancies.

When mycoplasma ascends the uterus, tubes, and ovaries, it results more often than either chlamydia or gonorrhea in noticeable symptoms of fever and abdominal pain and tenderness—an acute PID syndrome similar to that of chlamydia but with less scarring. If untreated, it can cause infertility from scarring of the tubes and uterus, miscarriage, low birth-weight infants, ectopic pregnancy, and acute fever and widespread pelvic infection following abortion or delivery of a child.

The diagnosis and treatment of mycoplasma are similar to those of chlamydia. A swab of fluid from the cervix is sent to a lab for a culture test, then examined under a microscope. Because the diseases are so similar, many doctors have a chlamydia culture done at the same time in order to rule out that disease. The treatment is identical to chlamydia treatment.

CHAPTER SIX

Cervical Infections, Endometritis, and Pelvic Inflammatory Disease

Gonorrhea, chlamydia, and mycoplasma, as we have seen, are not always simple diseases affecting only the cervix. Untreated, they cause an ascending disease syndrome. It is "ascending" because the first site of infection is usually the cervix, the gateway to the upper pelvic organs, where the infection causes **mucopurulent cervicitis**. From the cervix the infection spreads upwards to the endometrium or uterine lining, resulting in **endometritis** or inflammation. When the infection has spread to the fallopian tubes, ovaries, and

FIGURE 4:
The Female Reproductive Tract

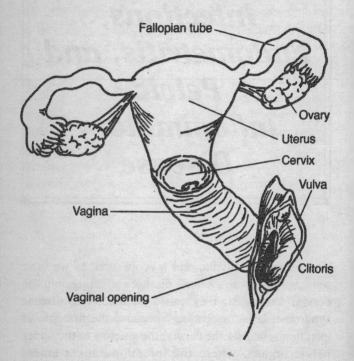

tissues of the upper pelvic organs in general, it is called **pelvic inflammatory disease.** Gonorrhea, chlamydia, and mycoplasma all cause similar symptoms and have the same general effect at each site; the differences are mostly in the severity of illness.

The ascending infection of the upper genital tract leading to pelvic inflammatory disease (PID) has been the most common sexually transmitted syndrome affecting women for two decades. Today the incidence of the PID syndrome is rising so fast that doctors now regard it as a secondary epidemic within the larger epidemic of the STDs that cause PID.

PID is especially dangerous because it is the most common cause of reproductive and infertility problems. The infections of the cervix, uterus, fallopian tubes, and ovaries can cause miscarriage, ectopic or tubal pregnancy (which is life-threatening and requires surgery), and illness in the newborn. It can affect long-term fertility by blocking and scarring both tubes and uterus.

Infections of the Cervix

Muco-purulent cervicitis, the name applied to common cervical infection, means inflammation of the cervix. When gonorrhea, chlamydia, and mycoplasma invade the vagina through sexual contact, they settle in the smooth lining cells of the cervix. The herpes simplex virus also causes such inflammation, but without pus. These STDs are more likely to infect the cervix rather than the vagina because the cervix provides a more favorable environment for their growth.

After infection these organisms produce a discharge from the duct at the center of the endocervix and cause **erythema,** or irritated redness. The cervix can be so inflamed that it bleeds from the slightest trauma, a condition known as **friability.**

Whereas gonorrhea and chlamydia cause inflammation and pus formation, herpes causes ulceration—the sores of this disease cover the cervix in nearly eighty percent of women who are having their initial attack. The sores usually heal without treatment and do not usually recur with subsequent attacks. Women with herpes ulcerations on the cervix or who are shedding herpes will have an abnormal Pap test showing **cervical atypia**—a change in the surface cells of the cervix associated with repeated irritation. Usually the atypia will disappear as the sores heal after the initial attack, though occasionally the atypia will persist. Cervical atypia can progress to a condition called **dysplasia,** which involves more drastic changes in the cells and is regarded as a precancerous condition.

Muco-purulent cervicitis (from gonorrhea, chlamydia, and mycoplasma) and herpes cervicitis (if no painful genital sore occurs) are painless, and the discharge is often mistaken for normal vaginal secretions. Occasionally a woman will experience light bleeding, but in general, cervicitis has no symptoms unless the disease responsible has also settled in the urethra, causing painful and frequent urination. As noted in the previous chapter, it is often only after a male partner develops the symptoms that a woman goes to the doctor and is diagnosed and treated for the underlying infection.

During a pelvic exam using a speculum it is easy for a doctor to make a diagnosis of cervical infection. She will see the discharge in the endocervix; the cervix itself will appear reddened and inflamed; and there may be bleeding and friability. The doctor will take a sample of the discharge for microscopic examination, looking for the presence of white cells the body produces to fight infection. Once the diagnosis is made, further tests are performed to identify which disease underlies the infection. When the underlying disease is treated—penicillin given by injection for gonorrhea, for example—the infection is killed and the cervix will heal itself.

If you have been diagnosed with cervicitis, it is likely your partner may be infected as well, even if he shows no symptoms. Men can harbor chlamydia and mycoplasma in their urethras often without ever developing symptoms. If they don't get treatment, they may reinfect you and others.

Three things that can make an infection established in the cervix (causing cervicitis) ascend into the pelvic organs are:

- an IUD: The IUD is treated as a foreign object by your body, creating an environment in which gonorrhea, chlamydia, and mycoplasma are highly likely to cause PID.
- surgical procedure: Having a dilatation and curettage (D&C), abortion, IUD insertion, or any kind of pelvic surgical procedure can introduce the disease organisms into the uterus where they can cause PID.

- menstruation: Gonorrhea can flare up into PID during menstruation.
- douching: This can push cervical infections into the upper reproductive tract. Don't douche unless directed by your doctor.

Endometritis

The endometrium—the lining of the uterus—connects at its base to the endocervix and to the fallopian tubes from each side. **Endometritis** is the inflammation of this lining from infection. Surgical procedures like abortion and Caesarean-section childbirth can cause a previously "silent" case of endometritis to develop into a full-blown PID syndrome. Common STDs like gonorrhea, chlamydia, and mycoplasma (and more rarely gardnerella) are more often responsible.

Sexually transmitted endometritis is the direct result of untreated muco-purulent cervicitis. The disease takes different forms: It can occur alone or as part of a general PID syndrome where the tubes and ovaries are infected as well. Symptoms may occur shortly after infection or months later and can be so mild as to go unnoticed or severe enough to require hospitalization.

When endometritis infection is severe, it causes acute illness: fever and intense abdominal pain, vaginal bleeding, and a foul-smelling vaginal discharge. During an examination an infected woman notices tenderness of the uterus and has a high white cell count signaling massive infection.

In milder sexually transmitted cases the symptoms are not as severe. They include vaginal discharge and bleeding and abdominal cramps. In fact, STD-related cases of endometritis are more likely to have no symptoms at all. This is doubly dangerous, since a silent infection may go on to cause damage to and scarring of the endometrium. Even your doctor may not find tenderness or other symptoms during a pelvic exam. When the endometrium is scarred, the fertilized embryo may not be able to find endometrial tissue healthy enough to attach itself to before developing further. The underlying disease can also lurk in the uterine lining, infecting the fetus either during pregnancy (when it can cause miscarriage) or during the actual passage through the birth canal at delivery.

The diagnosis of endometritis is not as simple as in muco-purulent cervicitis because, though cervicitis precedes endometritis, a test for any underlying disease might be negative if the bacteria have retreated from the cervix and are no longer present there. The diagnosis is usually made by relating symptoms to medical history. If a woman is experiencing pelvic pain and knows or thinks she has been exposed to an STD, has a new sex partner, or has undergone a surgical procedure that might have caused the endometritis, the doctor will want to perform tests to determine the underlying infectious organism and the extent of infection and damage by taking a tissue sample from the endometrium (endometrial biopsy).

Treatment depends on the severity of the disease. Acute infection often requires intravenous antibiotics, which are administered in a hospital, as well as sophisticated tests (like sonograms), performed usually only in hospitals or X-ray facilities. As in cervicitis, the underlying disease organism is treated with antibiotics. (See the cervicitis section for a description of methods of treatment for each cause.)

Cervicitis, Endometritis, and Pregnancy

Cervicitis and endometritis are dangerous for pregnant women because the underlying STD infection can be reactivated by surgical procedures like Caesarean section, and even normal delivery, causing massive infection. The underlying STD can also infect the baby (see gonorrhea and chlamydia sections for how they affect newborns). Cervicitis and endometritis can also cause miscarriage, infertility, and low-birth-weight infants. Many of the antibiotics used to combat these infections can't be used during pregnancy, which makes treatment more difficult.

Pelvic Inflammatory Disease (PID)

Pelvic inflammatory disease (PID) is an infection of the uterus and fallopian tubes. Most cases of PID in the U.S. each year—and most of the infections of the cervix and endometrium—are the result of STDs, and the major culprits are gonorrhea, chlamydia, and mycoplasma. Other common, nonsexually transmitted causes of PID are bacteria of the gut and vagina (like the bacteria responsible for vaginitis). A woman can have several STDs at the same time, as we saw with gonorrhea and chlamydia in the previous chapter, which occur together more than half the time. This combined infection makes diagnosis and treatment more complicated.

Acute PID

PID can be acute, and infection will rapidly set into the endometrium, fallopian tubes, and ovaries, and can spread throughout the entire pelvis and sometimes the entire abdomen. There will be tenderness of the pelvic organs in addition to scattered abdominal pain, high fever, and foul-smelling, often blood-tinged vaginal discharge. Someone with acute PID will feel very ill. Hospitalization is usually required.

Most acute PID is caused by gonorrhea and chlamydia (singly or together) or bacteria of the gut. When gonorrhea or chlamydia is responsible, the onset of the disease often coincides with menstruation, when the flow of blood and shed tissue provides a pathway for the bacteria to ascend and a rich environment for their growth. Acute gonorrheal PID can develop quickly, three to five days after initial infection has set in in the cervix. Gonorrhea is also much more likely to cause the acute symptoms of fever, inflammation, vaginal discharge, and severe pain. Acute illness from chlamydia, however, can take up to three weeks from the time of infection to develop. Though chlamydia and mycoplasma are more often responsible for "silent PID," when either occurs together with gonorrhea, acute PID is often the result.

Silent PID

Years ago doctors began to notice that most of the women they saw with tubal damage and scarring could not remember having suffered any acute pelvic inflammation in the past. When cultures were taken from the fallopian tubes of these women, however, they showed evidence of previous infection with a variety of STDs. The conclusion: Pelvic infections can damage the reproductive tract without ever producing symptoms. Today we know that tubal infection without symptoms—silent PID—is much more common than acute PID. Most women suffering from infertility due to STDs have had this silent PID syndrome. Silent PID is particularly common from chlamydia infection.

Diagnosing PID

Acute PID is easily diagnosed. High fever, vaginal discharge, severe abdominal pain during a gynecological examination, and a high white blood cell count from a blood test all reveal the presence of massive abdominal infection. After ruling out endometriosis, ovarian cyst, acute appendicitis, and the various abdominal infections caused by intestinal problems, the doctor will probably admit a woman with acute PID to the hospital, where further tests will help reveal the extent of the disease and intravenous antibiotic treatment can begin immediately.

Silent PID, with no telltale symptoms, is much harder to diagnose. The circumstances, either singly or in combination, under which a doctor might suspect silent PID are:

- inability to conceive after one year of intercourse without birth control
- unexplained tubal pregnancy or multiple miscarriages

- infection following surgical procedure or childbirth cervicitis or endometritis
- unexplained urinary tract symptoms, arthritis, or abdominal pain
- use of intrauterine device (IUD) for birth control
- multiple sex partners and prior history of STDs (because women who have had other STDs are more likely to have tubal damage)
- being sexually active and of adolescent age

After a preliminary diagnosis is made, the doctor will want to test definitively for the organism underlying the infection. First, cervical secretions are cultured and examined for STDs like gonorrhea and chlamydia. Sometimes, however, the infection, having settled in the tubes, is no longer present in the cervix, and tests will be negative. In such cases a laparoscopy might be performed, allowing the doctor to see the pelvic organs and fallopian tubes and sample tissue.

What Happens during a PID Episode

When the invading disease organism reaches the endometrium from the cervix, subsequent infection of the fallopian tubes—and hence PID—is likely. Because your body does not build sufficient immunity to gonorrhea or chlamydia during an initial attack, each time you're exposed again the likelihood of pelvic infection resulting in infertility increases. Once the infection is in the tubes, the body's immune system attacks the disease organisms in what is known as an acute inflammatory response. White blood cells mass at the site of infection, engulfing and digesting the invaders. This mass, however, may also temporarily block the tube.

After the infection subsides, the body heals the "wound" at the site of infection by laying down strands of fibrous scar tissue. Since the diameter of the fallopian tubes is so small, even the slightest irregularity of their smooth lining—and scar tissue *is* coarse and uneven—can hamper the passage of the egg. When the disease is in the initial inflammatory stage, the tube can be blocked entirely, preventing both fertilization and passage of the egg.

Effects of PID on the Body

Infertility and Ectopic Pregnancy

When the tubes become blocked either from acute infection or from scarring, conception, in which egg meets sperm in the fallopian tube, is made more difficult. Unfortunately, about one fifth of all women who have had acute PID at least once will be infertile from such scarring. With each episode of PID the chances of infertility increase.

Ectopic pregnancy, in which the fertilized egg implants itself in any place other than the uterus, is another complication resulting directly from PID, and one that has been increasing markedly over the last twenty years. In ectopic pregnancy the fertilized ovum gets lost in the webs of scar tissue in the tubes and implants itself there. Eventually, a tubal pregnancy will rupture the narrow tube. This is a serious medical emergency in which the woman experiences acute abdominal pain, bleeding, and fever from the infection that follows.

If undiagnosed, a ruptured tubal pregnancy can

cause death from shock and massive bleeding. The death of the embryo also almost always occurs. Even if diagnosed, such a rupture can cause irreversible damage to the tubes and subsequent infertility.

Pelvic Abscess

Some women with PID, especially those who use the IUD, develop a **pelvic abscess**—a pus-filled cavity—during an acute PID episode. The danger of such abscesses is not only that large ones must be surgically removed but also that they cause heavy pelvic scarring, which can contribute to later infertility. The infection commonly spreads throughout the abdomen and bloodstream.

Abdominal Infection and the Fitz Hugh Curtis Syndrome

In some women with acute PID the infection travels up from the tubes into the abdominal cavity, causing fever and infection of the other organs in the abdomen not usually affected by STDs, such as the liver, gall bladder, and appendix. Before discovering the source in an underlying sexually transmitted disease, doctors had difficulty diagnosing this condition. In some cases, of which the **Fitz Hugh Curtis syndrome** is one example, the infection settles in one organ, causing specific disease there. In the Fitz Hugh Curtis syndrome the disease organism attacks the liver, causing hepatitis or inflammation. Though this syndrome used to be thought to be caused solely by gonorrheal infections, today chlamydia is also recognized to cause it. Fitz Hugh Curtis syndrome mimics acute cholecystitis, or acute infection of the gallbladder, and before it was recognized and treated as a chlamydial infection some women had their gallbladders or appendixes removed unnecessarily.

Arthritis

Both chlamydia and gonorrhea can cause joint pain and swelling in ankles, wrists, and knees, or acute infectious arthritis. This condition is difficult to diagnose since the symptoms appear and disappear spontaneously. Acute infectious arthritis occurs when the original gonorrheal or chlamydial infection has spread beyond the pelvic region, firmly establishing itself in other parts of the body. Often, this type of arthritis is mistaken for other more common forms like rheumatoid arthritis, osteoarthritis, or joint injury.

Chronic Pelvic Pain

Some women who have had previous infections resulting in heavy fibrous scarring of the pelvic organs experience intense, constant pain in the pelvic region. Though not all women who have such heavy scarring suffer this kind of pain, doctors believe that the scarring—which can completely encase the tubes and ovaries and deform the endometrium—is responsible.

Treatment of PID

Since PID is the result of an underlying infection, it is only by treating that infection specifically that you halt the effects of the ongoing syndrome.

A woman with acute PID will experience high fever, tenderness, and great pain during the examination, and the doctor might decide that hospitalization for intensive treatment is best. This means you will have intravenous antibiotics (fed into a vein in your arm through an IV tube) and diagnostic tests to determine the extent of infection and damage. Not all cases—even those with pelvic pain—require hospitalization. That decision will be made by you and your doctor. In either case, the doctor will want to start treatment immediately, even before culture or blood test results are in.

In all cases of PID, bed rest for several weeks and pelvic rest (no sexual intercourse) are extremely important. This allows the pelvis to heal.

For more serious gonorrheal infection that has spread to the tubes but has not yet caused high fever or severe abdominal tenderness, the doctor may not choose hospitalization but may begin treatment with:

- one injection of *cefoxitin* (two grams) into muscle, plus *probenecid* injection (one gram), plus *doxycycline,* 100 milligrams taken orally twice daily for two weeks

or

- *ampicillin, amoxicillin,* or *ceftriaxone* in capsules for several weeks, accompanied by *tetracycline* or *doxycycline* for two weeks, with all doses determined by your doctor.

or

- *ampicillin* or *amoxicillin* by injection, given with *probenecid* and *doxycycline* by mouth or

- *procaine penicillin* injection taken with *probenecid* and *doxycycline* by mouth

or

- *ceftriaxone* injection, 250 milligrams injected into muscle at one site, plus *doxycycline* as above.

The treatment for mycoplasma-related PID, which commonly occurs together with either gonorrhea or chlamydia, is the same as treatment for either one alone. All of these treatments are general rather than precise. Although any treatment will probably involve one or more of the antibiotics above, your doctor will want to adjust treatment to fit your case. She may use other, similar treatments derived from her own experience.

After the symptoms of acute PID have subsided and the antibiotic treatment is complete, your doctor may want to assess the extent of the damage caused by the infection. One way to do this is to use a **sonogram,** which forms an image on a television screen by bouncing sound waves off a given area of the body. A sonogram can show if the infection has caused an abscess to form that may require surgery. Another method is the **laparoscopy,** which allows the doctor to examine the pelvic organs directly through a lighted lens inserted through a small incision in the abdomen.

If a woman has trouble getting pregnant or has chronic pain after having PID, there are other (surgical) treatments that can reverse the effects of PID scarring and the infertility such scarring can cause.

One such alternative is **tubal surgery,** in which the doctor first exposes the pelvic organs, then uses a scalpel to remove the clumps of scar tissue that may be blocking the tubes. In recent years, microsurgery—with fine instruments capable of removing very small amounts of tissue precisely and reconnecting the tubes—has helped many previously infertile women have children. Tubal surgery cannot be done, however, if the ends of the tubes near the ovaries are damaged, swollen, or scarred.

When tubes are extensively damaged or even ruptured after a tubal pregnancy, but at least five centimeters are disease-free, surgeons can reconstruct them in a procedure called **tubuloplasty.** Often a splint of Teflon will be inserted to take the place of part of the tube if the ovary end of the tube and its lining are intact. Though such modern technological advances are helping more and more women become fertile once again, these procedures are very expensive and have very low success rates (probably less than thirty percent in severe cases).

In vitro fertilization, in which an already-fertilized egg is surgically attached to the uterine lining, is often the best solution for women made infertile by PID.

Preventing PID

When a woman protects herself against sexually transmitted disease she is protecting herself against PID. Limiting the number of sexual partners reduces the chance of contracting PID. Women who use condoms, for example, have extremely low rates of PID. Other barrier contraceptives like the diaphragm also prevent common PID-causing STDs like gonorrhea, chlamydia, and mycoplasma from gaining entry to the cervix, the first step in the PID syndrome. Abandoning the IUD, which has been shown to be a major cause of all cervical and pelvic infections, in favor of one of these barrier forms of birth control is another positive preventive measure. Regular, yearly gynecological exams with a Pap smear and cervical cultures for chlamydia and gonorrhea will help catch an infection that might later develop into PID. Yearly exams are especially important since some cases of PID aren't sexually transmitted at all but need to be considered just as seriously and treated just as carefully. If you are not monogamous, routine cultures for gonorrhea and chlamydia should be done more frequently—ask your doctor.

Finally, don't douche. Douching can introduce cervical infections into the uterus and tubes and so should be done only when recommended by your doctor.

PART

IV

Acquired Immune Deficiency Syndrome (AIDS) and Other Viral STDs

The Human Immunodeficiency Virus (HIV) and Acquired Immune Deficiency Syndrome (AIDS)

What are HIV and AIDS?

Acquired Immune Deficiency Syndrome (AIDS) is a long-term, fatal viral disease that can be sexually transmitted. It is caused by the **human immunodeficiency virus (HIV),** which systematically invades and destroys the human immune system that normally protects us from the infectious organisms we come into contact with every day. When HIV has so weakened the immune system that the body can no longer fight back, the person gets what are called **opportunistic infections**

like pneumonia, tuberculosis, and Kaposi's sarcoma (a formerly rare kind of cancer). At this point they are said to have AIDS.

Opportunistic infections get their name from the fact that many of the organisms that cause them are around us—in the air, in the food we eat—all the time. These common organisms don't cause disease in people with normal immune systems because our bodies fight them off quickly and efficiently. People with AIDS usually have very poorly functioning immune systems and thus contract disease more easily.

Each infection further weakens a person with AIDS and leaves him or her less able to fight the next one. When people die of AIDS, it is one of these opportunistic infections that, in most cases, is directly responsible for their death. AIDS, though it may take as long as ten years for its symptoms to develop, is invariably fatal, and as of today there is no treatment that cures it.

What is the difference between having AIDS and being infected with HIV?

HIV is the virus that causes AIDS. AIDS itself is at one end of the range of HIV infection and describes a particular medical situation in which the immune system functions poorly, if at all. Doctors say people have AIDS when they have measurable levels of antibodies to the virus in their blood, when they have swollen lymph nodes all over the body, and when they develop one of the opportunistic infections that signal total immune breakdown. People who are described as being HIV-positive, on the other hand, are at the other, mild end of the spectrum and merely have a measurable level of antibodies to the virus in their bloodstream as a result of being exposed to it. (An AIDS test is testing for antibodies to the virus in the bloodstream.) People who are HIV-positive may appear and feel healthy and have no symptoms, but some, perhaps the majority, will go on to develop full-blown AIDS with all the symptoms within ten years of first being exposed.

How does HIV attack the immune system?

One of the most basic parts of the immune system is the lymphocyte, a kind of white blood cell that has the ability to recognize invading infectious organisms and to stimulate the body's production of antibodies that combat such infections. There are different kinds of lymphocytes, each with a specific purpose. "T" lymphocytes, for example, fight off infections cell-to-cell; they migrate to a specific site of infection and literally surround and absorb the infectious cell to destroy it. Other "B" lymphocytes (or "B" cells) have a larger range, producing antibodies that circulate throughout the bloodstream to fight infection there.

There are different kinds of T cells, but only two of them—the T_4 and T_8 cells—concern us here. T_4 cells are also called "helper cells"; they are like the quarterback on a football team. T_4 cells have a particular ability to recognize invading infectious cells and then call plays to direct the other specialized white blood cells in the best way to overcome the infectious cells.

T_8 cells, also called "killer" cells, are more like lone rangers, killing the infectious invaders independently without necessarily activating other cells.

What HIV does is to slowly but steadily deplete the body's supply of T_4 cells—the quarterbacks—so that the body is no longer able to fight off infectious organisms common in the environment like viruses, fungi, parasites, and bacteria like tuberculosis. Eventually, the number of T_4 cells declines to the point where the normal ratio of more T_4 to T_8 reverses, with T_8 cells dominating. It is at this point that the immune system breaks down almost completely, leaving the person vulnerable to various opportunistic infections that characterize the syndrome called AIDS.

HIV is so deadly because the virus overpowers the immune system by taking over the normal cell reproduction process. All cells constantly reproduce themselves according to a genetic blueprint. HIV is a retrovirus, which means it has the unusual ability to insert itself into the genetic blueprint of the cell it invades. When that cell reproduces itself, it also reproduces new particles of the virus. Every time the T cell reproduces it will reproduce a copy of the virus, too, until the T cell dies. Those copies will leave the cell and attack other healthy cells.

In AIDS, this happens millions and millions of times all over the body, not just in lymphocytes but in similar cells in the bone marrow and intestines, and perhaps other areas as well. All of the newly copied virus particles spill out of the cell into the bloodstream. The symptoms are not initially present because it takes HIV a long time to destroy the immune system. This is called the latent stage. The latent stage occurs from the time the person contracts HIV until the time he develops objective evidence of immune breakdown. It can last from several months to more than ten years. Throughout the entire course of the latent stage, more and more healthy cells are being invaded and destroyed by HIV.

Generally, for the first several years after becoming infected with the HIV virus the body does its best to fight off the infection by producing antibodies and by the actions of the killer lymphocyte cells. Someone who is HIV-positive has these antibodies in his or her blood, and this is what an AIDS test is testing for. It is when the number of T_4 cells drops below normal—as the HIV takes over more and more of these lymphocyte cells—that the body becomes susceptible to opportunistic infection. When a person has such an infection, he or she is said to have AIDS. Specifically, a medical diagnosis of AIDS is made if a person is HIV-positive, has had swollen lymph nodes for a certain amount of time, and has an opportunistic infection like Kaposi's sarcoma or pneumocystis carinii.

How is HIV transmitted by sex?

The particles of HIV circulate freely in the blood but mostly live in lymphocytes, which are present in most body fluids, like semen, blood, cervical and vaginal secretions, saliva, even urine, and tears. Any activity or behavior that brings an infected person's body fluids into contact with yours (called "an exchange of bodily fluids") can transmit the virus to you, though how likely you are to get the disease depends on the particular fluid and other factors. Most people get HIV through exposure to infected blood, semen, and vaginal or cervical secretions, and, in this country, such exposure and infection have happened mostly through sexual contact. Today, however, it appears that the largest number of new cases are from IV drug use.

What does it mean to say a certain kind of sexual activity is "risky"?

In the next few pages you'll learn how specific ways of having sex can lead to one partner giving HIV to the other, and exactly why each is risky. They run from most risky (anal intercourse) to least risky (deep kissing where saliva is exchanged). But saying a certain kind of sexual behavior is "least risky" is like saying only some guns are dangerous. All guns can kill people, and all kinds of sexual behavior in which your body fluids come into contact with an infected person's can lead to your getting HIV. Remember as you read this that all of these kinds of sexual behavior can transmit HIV, and that the least risky only means that transmission is less likely, *not* impossible.

Why is anal sex so risky?

Having anal intercourse, especially being the receptive or passive partner (as all women are), is the number one riskiest sexual activity. The anus is lined with thin and delicate tissue with blood vessels lying close to the skin. When a man ejaculates during anal intercourse, his semen comes into direct contact with the thin tissue lining the rectum of the passive partner. Virus particles can gain access to the bloodstream through this thin tissue and cause infection. Since the anus is small and the tissue so fragile, the entrance and movement of the penis can make tiny tears in the skin of the rectum, providing an easy entrance for the virus where the underlying tissue is exposed and small blood vessels are broken.

Though the risk of anal intercourse is higher for the receptive partner, the active partner who inserts his penis can also become infected through the mucous membrane tissue at the tip of the penis, which is very vulnerable. Passive or active, anal intercourse is responsible for the largest number of HIV infections in the U.S., with most cases in male homosexuals. *Anyone* who has anal intercourse with an HIV carrier (someone infected with the virus) has a great risk of getting the disease.

How risky is vaginal intercourse?

Most women who are infected with HIV contracted it through *vaginal* intercourse with men who got it originally from contaminated hypodermic needles or other drug equipment while injecting drugs like heroin or cocaine into their veins. Vaginal intercourse with an infected man is the most risky sexual activity after anal sex. When a man ejaculates inside a woman's vagina, the semen comes into contact with the delicate tissue of the endocervix. Since this tissue has many blood vessels near its surface, the virus can easily gain access to the bloodstream. It is also possible, though less likely, that the semen can get into the bloodstream through the vaginal walls and mucous membranes of the vulva as well.

Men can also be infected with HIV during vaginal intercourse from contact with the vaginal and cervical secretions of a woman who has HIV. This is not as likely, however, since studies have shown that semen contains many more lymphocytes (which harbor the virus) than vaginal secretions. Women, in fact, are much more likely to get HIV from an infected partner via oral sex and vaginal intercourse than men for this reason. Men and women have the same risk of getting HIV if they are the passive partners in anal sex.

How about foreplay?

All kinds of sexual foreplay—fondling or caressing each other's genitals, a man stimulating a woman's genitals with his hands or the head of his penis, a woman stimulating a man with her hands, embracing and cuddling intimately while naked—can also transmit HIV when any exchange of fluids occurs, though the risk is less than that of vaginal intercourse. Such an exchange could occur if the semen your partner ejaculates (or the few drops that reach the tip of the penis before ejaculation) reaches the moist mucous membranes of your vulva or vagina. Or, if it is on his pubic hair, the semen can reach your vulva when you embrace or rub against each other. A man could get HIV from a woman's vaginal secretions when he touches her and then himself, or even by her rubbing her vulva against the head of his penis. As with vaginal intercourse, however, the risk for a man is lower, since fewer HIV-carrying lymphocytes are present in vaginal and cervical secretions.

What about oral sex?

Men and women can get HIV from oral sex, though no case has been reliably proved to have been transmitted only through oral sex. Still, it is possible for a woman to get HIV from a man when his infected semen penetrates the mucous membranes of her mouth when he ejaculates. The mouth has a large blood supply with many blood vessels the virus can penetrate. A man performing oral sex on a woman is less likely to get HIV if she's a carrier because her vaginal and cervical fluids have fewer of the lymphocytes that carry the disease, and because most contact is between the mouth and clitoris rather than the well-lubricated vaginal walls or cervix.

If a man or woman with HIV is performing oral sex on a partner, it is also possible that the infected person's saliva, which contains HIV-carrying lymphocytes, could infect the partner through the tip of the penis or the mucous membranes of the vulva and vagina. Again, it is almost impossible to pinpoint oral sex as the cause of transmission, since those with HIV who have been studied have also had intercourse and engaged in other kinds of sexual behavior with an infected partner.

What about "rimming" (mouth-to-anus contact) and "watersports" (when one partner urinates into the other's anus or vagina)?

Because HIV is present in the feces, mouth-to-anus contact can transmit HIV. "Watersports"—any activity in which one partner's urine comes into contact with the other's bodily fluids—can be risky, too, for both partners. All of these kinds of sexual activity can be very risky, and you should avoid them.

Can HIV be transmitted through kissing, in saliva?

The answer is yes—possibly. HIV has been found, in very small quantities, in the lymphocytes in saliva, but not all those infected have HIV in their saliva, and even in those who do, HIV is not present at all times. It is possible that open-mouthed, "deep," or French kissing, in which saliva is exchanged in a much larger amount than when kissing on the lips, can transmit HIV. Casual kissing—on the lips, cheek, face, neck, etc.—that does not involve saliva exchange *does not* transmit HIV.

Can a mother pass it on to her child, in the womb or through breast-feeding?

Yes. Since large numbers of the lymphocytes that carry HIV are present in the blood, pregnant mothers can pass HIV on to their unborn children in the womb. This happens because the mother's blood circulation is shared with the fetus's, so virus particles in her blood also circulate into the fetal blood system. An infected mother has, in fact, more than a fifty percent chance of transmitting HIV to her unborn. There is also evidence that a mother can give HIV to her child through breast-feeding, probably from contact between the infant's mouth and the mucous membranes of the mother's nipples.

Can you get HIV without having sex?

Blood transfusion, in which one person's blood is fed directly into the veins of another, is another way people get HIV. About three percent of all AIDS cases are due to blood tranfusion, though since 1985 all blood donors and the blood they give are tested for HIV infection. Now it is *very* unlikely that you will get HIV from a transfusion. Before April 1985, about 1 in 400 blood donations was HIV-positive, which means anyone who received a transfusion in the years prior to that is at some risk. Contaminated blood is highly contagious, and one transfusion is often enough to transmit HIV. It is thought that most of those who were infected through transfusion before blood bank AIDS testing have already become ill.

Hemophiliacs who receive transfusions of clotting factors (which are collected from a pool of donors) run a higher risk of contracting HIV than the recipients of standard blood transfusions.

How do IV drug users get HIV?

Contaminated blood is also the way most intravenous (IV) drug users get HIV. The virus is passed through shared needles, syringes, and "cookers" (used to dissolve the heroin or cocaine into a liquid). The virus can live for several days in the tiny drops of blood left in needles and syringes, infecting anyone who uses them.

Is there any other way women can get HIV?

There is also some evidence that women who receive artificial insemination from anonymous donors in order to become pregnant could be exposed through semen from HIV-carrying donors. If you are considering artificial insemination, you should make sure the sperm bank or fertility clinic you are using tests all donations for HIV.

Ear piercing and tattoos are also mentioned as possible, though *unproven,* ways HIV can be transmitted.

What are some of the myths about getting AIDS?

There are many myths about getting HIV and AIDS. You *cannot* get AIDS or HIV from casual contact with an HIV-positive person. Casual contact means talking, shaking hands, breathing the same air, getting coughed on or sneezed on, eating food they prepare, or sharing a meal; it includes hugging or touching or even casual kissing that does not involve saliva exchange. You *don't* get HIV or AIDS from living in the same house, from being around an infected person when he or she is sick, from being in the same schoolroom, or from sharing clothing or towels. You *don't* get AIDS from insect bites, either.

Good evidence for all of this comes from studies of families of AIDS victims, who have daily contact in all the ways above, and in studies of health care workers like doctors, nurses, lab technicians, and hospital personnel who care for AIDS patients daily. Though health care workers have a slightly higher risk of getting HIV than the general population, some of that risk can be traced to accidents—a nurse who sticks himself with a "dirty" needle accidentally or a lab tech who splashes herself with HIV-contaminated blood. Since these people come into contact with AIDS-contaminated body fluids like blood, semen, feces, and saliva every day, if there were a risk from casual contact many, many more health care workers would already have been infected.

What is a high-risk group, and what are the high-risk groups for HIV and AIDS?

"High-risk group" is a term used to describe individuals who share a particular behavior or behaviors that make it more likely that they will contract a given disease because of that behavior. High-risk groups for HIV and AIDS infection include:

- IV drug users, who can also infect their lovers and unborn children.
- homosexual men, who run a high HIV risk because of sexual practices like anal intercourse.

- bisexual men, who often have sex with homosexual men as well as with women.
- hemophiliacs and other people who received blood transfusions before 1985, when universal screening for HIV was first adopted.
- male and female prostitutes, who often sell sex to support their drug habit—both of which expose them to HIV. Male prostitutes run an even higher risk because they practice anal intercourse with homosexual men, another high-risk group.
- people who have multiple sex partners. This increases their risk of getting HIV because with each new partner they are exposed to all of his or her previous partners, one of whom may have been infected. If you have sex with three people in a year, you've been exposed directly to them, but you've also been indirectly exposed to the people they had sex with (or were exposed to through others) before you. If you begin to count, the number of indirect contacts climbs pretty quickly, even if you've only had sex with three people.

How can I figure out my own risk of getting HIV through sex?

If you are not in any of the risk groups above, your risk of getting HIV generally depends on three things: who your partner is, what you do with him or her, and how often you do it.

Having a heterosexual encounter with a man who you know has been bisexual in the past, for example, means you, in effect, are being exposed to all his previous lovers, male and female, through him. You run a further risk in what you do: Vaginal or anal intercourse without a condom or use of nonoxynol-9 (a sperm-killing chemical that is somewhat effective in killing HIV) could expose you if he is a carrier. Oral sex with a condom, foreplay, and masturbating each other—generally safe sex—don't provide the exchange of body fluids necessary for transmission and so are much less risky, no matter what your lover's past sexual history is. Each time you have unprotected intercourse with him or engage in any other activity that involves the exchange of fluids, you're increasing the chance for transmission. Evidence for this has been seen in wives of hemophiliacs and wives of IV drug users. When their husbands are HIV-positive, these women are from ten to seventy percent more likely to get HIV within several years of their husbands' infection if they have steady sexual relations with them.

What if I'm monogamous and had only one lover for a long time?

The general rule of thumb for heterosexuals is that if you and your partner have been monogamous for ten years and aren't exposed through any other of the risk factors (you aren't a hemophiliac or IV drug user, for example), then you have no risk of getting HIV from sex.

Can you get HIV more easily from someone who has had it longer?

Yes. The longer a person has been infected, the more infectious that person is. Though the body's immune system attempts to control the infection, as time goes on the virus takes over more and more lymphocytes, and more free viral particles are released into the bloodstream, making all body fluids more virus-laden and therefore infectious. The speed of this process varies from person to person, since each responds to the HIV infection differently. In fact, there is no way even for a doctor to tell how long someone has been infected with HIV. Long before someone gets acutely ill with AIDS (when the immune system is no longer functioning at all), all his or her body fluids—blood, semen, cervical/vaginal secretions, saliva, etc.—may be highly infectious. People with HIV will remain capable of infecting others for the rest of their lives.

If I've been exposed to someone who has HIV, does that mean I have it, too?

No. Being exposed—when you have exchanged bodily fluids with an HIV carrier during intercourse, for example—does not necessarily mean that the infection was passed on to you. Whether or not you get it depends on how you are exposed, how often, and other factors that still aren't completely understood. HIV must have a portal of entry to the body, that is, it must gain access to the bloodstream either directly via a blood vessel or indirectly through a mucous membrane. Some activities, like anal intercourse, transmit

HIV "better" than others. That's why anal sex is "most risky" and oral sex "less risky."

Individuals differ in the way their bodies work; they have different body chemistry and are exposed to different diseases. These variables may account for why one person gets HIV from a single exposure while another does not. One woman might have vaginal intercourse with an HIV-positive man once and get HIV, while another woman only gets HIV after months of exposure through vaginal intercourse.

One factor that does increase a woman's chances of getting HIV, if exposed, is having genital sores. These openings in the surface tissue of the vulva, vagina, or cervix (or on or around the penis, in men) provide easy access for HIV. In Africa, where such sores and the STDs that cause them are common, heterosexuals are just as likely to get HIV as any other group, and it is thought that genital sores may be part of the cause.

Any infection that causes inflammation of the cervix also creates an environment where HIV transmission is more likely, since the lymphocytes the virus prefers are always present at such sites of infection. Most of the common STDs like gonorrhea, chlamydia, and herpes cause cervical inflammation.

What are the symptoms of HIV infection?

HIV infection is generally divided into six stages, though it may be as long as five or six years before any serious symptoms are experienced. The stages run from stage 0 (initial infection) to stage 6 (full-blown

AIDS). Some people never get the initial flulike symptoms and only discover they have AIDS after getting an initial opportunistic infection that signals the weakening of the immune system.

Stage 0 usually lasts several months but can be as long as a year; it is the time from initial infection to when antibodies can be detected with a blood test. At this time the virus is attacking lymphocytes, and the body is beginning to produce antibodies to fight it. There are generally no symptoms, and the infected individual looks and feels healthy.

In Stage 1, antibodies to the virus can be detected in the blood. Symptoms at this point may but don't always include a temporary flulike illness resembling mononucleosis, with symptoms of fever, swollen lymph glands, and a mild, red, blotchy rash that lasts several days, and often these symptoms may not be noticed at all. Sometimes a person in this stage will also have neurological symptoms that show the virus has invaded the brain and central nervous system. This is, however, unusual. These symptoms range from mild headaches to drowsiness, neck stiffness, muscle rigidity, and seizures when inflammation of the brain occurs. All of these symptoms will eventually disappear.

Stage 1 usually begins within a year after initial infection and lasts from three to eight months. Most people still feel healthy, and not everyone gets the flulike and neurological symptoms.

The distinguishing symptom of Stage 2 is swollen lymph glands throughout the body, and for many people this is the first sign of disease. An HIV-infected person would feel hard, swollen lumps—the lymph glands—in the neck underneath the chin, at the sides of the throat, and sometimes around the collarbone. These lumps may also be felt under the arms and in the groin. These swollen glands are usually not painful, but they may feel tender if pressed.

During Stage 2, which is an incubation period lasting from three to five years, the infected person usually still feels and looks healthy. It is during this time, however, that the virus is doing serious damage to the body's immune system, slowly invading and taking over infection-fighting T_4 helper lymphocytes.

Stages 3, 4, and 5 are usually treated as a whole because they share symptoms, and exactly when those symptoms will appear is hard to gauge. At this stage the immune system has broken down to the point where it can be detected with something called a skin test, though the person doesn't feel there's anything wrong. In a skin test the doctor injects small amounts of foreign substances (like yeast) into the skin. Normally, the body recognizes these as foreign substances and produces small red bumps on the surface of the skin where they were injected. In the HIV-infected person in these stages, however, there is no response, since the T_4 helper cells—which would normally recognize these substances as foreign and show this by an immune response (raising a bump on the skin)—have been invaded and made useless by the HIV.

Usually the first evidence of immune breakdown is **thrush,** an infection caused by the yeast candida, which infects the mucous membranes of the throat and tongue. Thrush looks like white spots and reddish sores on the tongue and in the throat and causes a persistently sore throat and trouble swallowing. (Yeast is almost always present in the intestines of healthy men, and in the vagina as well as the intestines of healthy women. Normally, the body's immune system keeps it in check.) In women, getting a vaginal yeast infection alone, *without getting thrush* in the throat at the same time, is almost never related to HIV infection.

The number of T_4 cells available to help fight infection continues to decline in stages 3, 4, and 5, leaving the body defenseless against other infections of the mucous membranes. The recurrence of herpes simplex sores around the anus, vagina, penis, and mouth is common. Some people have fuzzy white particles on the tongue that can't be rubbed off, though why these occur is not known. In addition, lymph gland enlargement will progress and the person may begin to feel tired and run-down and may also lose weight. These stages can last from three to five years (average three years) before the onset of Stage 6, which is full-blown AIDS itself.

What are the symptoms of AIDS?

Stage 6 of HIV infection (which usually occurs a year or two after entering Stage 5) is full-blown AIDS. AIDS occurs when the immune system no longer functions at all. While in the previous stage of HIV infection opportunistic infections attacked the external mucous membranes, in Stage 6 infectious organisms that would be harmless to the healthy person cause serious illness and ravage whole body systems.

This systematic opportunistic infection is not HIV but is caused by what HIV does to the immune system. There are thousands of disease organisms that can and do attack the body in this stage of HIV, though here we will look only at those most common in the U.S. Such infections can be caused by bacteria, fungi, viruses, and parasites, and they range from the commonplace to the exotic. AIDS patients often have several opportunistic infections at once, sometimes affecting the same organ or body system. It is the constant attack of infection after infection that eventually weakens the body to the point where the person with AIDS dies, usually from complications caused by being ill for so long with so many things rather than due to any single infection.

What opportunistic infections do most people with AIDS get?

Most often, opportunistic infections attack particular systems: the lungs, the nervous system, the skin, and the gastrointestinal tract.

All infections of the lungs cause symptoms like shortness of breath, coughing, chest pain, high fever, and the accumulation of phlegm. As the infection attacks the lining of the lungs, the lungs work less efficiently, providing less oxygen in the blood. When a person with such a lung infection can no longer breathe unaided, a respirator, which breathes for them, may help. Some patients die within days, others after several weeks, even if the underlying infection is promptly and properly treated.

Although many different kinds of infections cause pneumonia in AIDS patients, the most common are **pneuocystis carinii pneumonia (PCP), cytomegalovirus (CMV), tuberculosis, cryptococcus neoformans, and herpes simplex virus.**

Pneumocystis carinii pneumonia (PCP), caused by a single-cell protozoon, is one of the most common lung infections in AIDS patients and was the first to be associated with AIDS. Until 1981, when many cases of PCP began to appear in homosexuals with AIDS, PCP was a disease usually found only in elderly people with immune systems destroyed by cancer and newborns still developing an immune system. Its symptoms include fever, difficulty in breathing, dry cough, and a characteristic appearance of the lungs on a chest X ray.

Cytomegalovirus (CMV) causes pneumonia in AIDS patients (as well as intestinal and brain infections), with the same symptoms as PCP. Often CMV appears with another infection like Kaposi's sarcoma. CMV can also infect the brain and cause blindness.

Tuberculosis, a bacterium common in the environment, used to be epidemic. It was wiped out largely through better sanitation and health standards but today has reappeared as a major cause of pneumonia in people with AIDS. Some AIDS patients are found to have gotten pneumonia from typical tuberculosis bacteria (those that cause infection in the general population), which suggests that it is a reactivation of tuberculosis they had had long before, but which their then-healthy immune system had kept in check. Atypical tuberculosis bacteria—exotic and very rare varieties—are usually seen only in AIDS patients, showing how vulnerable such people are to any exposure to infection.

Cryptococcus neoformans is a fungus that does not usually cause disease in people with healthy immune systems. In people with AIDS this fungus causes pneumonia as well as meningitis. Legionella, the same bacteria that causes Legionnaire's disease, can result in pneumonia and meningitis in AIDS patients. The herpes simplex virus can also cause pneumonia in AIDS patients.

When people with AIDS get these and other lung infections, the course of their pneumonia is often unpredictable. Some people don't survive their first attack of PCP, while others may survive many attacks over several years. Often, more than one infection is involved, which makes the pneumonia not only more difficult to fight, but also more severe in its consequences.

The conditions described above are only the most common causes of lung disease in AIDS patients. All are devastating only because HIV has made the person unable to fight off the everyday infectious organisms that do not affect individuals with healthy immune systems.

The brain and spinal cord, which together make up the nervous system, are frequent sites of opportunistic infection. Such infections are difficult to diagnose and treat because doctors can't take specimens for testing to isolate a particular organism as easily as they do with other internal organs. The brain is encased in bone and skin, and the spinal cord in the vertebrae, making biopsy (tissue sampling) difficult. In addition, the nervous system is more fragile and is directly responsible for controlling the other systems of the body. This is why infections of the nervous system can and do kill people with AIDS very quickly. General symptoms of many of these infections are headache, neck stiffness, memory loss, personality changes, seizures, and even coma.

Sometimes brain infection can cause a condition known as "AIDS dementia" in which a person can undergo severe personality changes and be irritable, confused, and overly sensitive to noise. Doctors believe that the virus itself may also cause AIDS dementia.

The same organisms, from bacteria to fungi, that cause lung disease also cause nervous system disease in people with AIDS. In addition to cryptococcus, herpes simplex, and tuberculosis, toxoplasmosis is a common source of infections. Toxoplasmosis is a protozoal parasite found in many cats. Although the disease can be caught by healthy people, too, in people with AIDS it can cause blindness, meningitis (spinal cord infection), and brain masses that put pressure on the brain and spinal cord leading to paralysis, coma, and sometimes death.

Opportunistic infections also attack the gastrointestinal tract (the stomach and intestines) of many of those who have AIDS. Cryptococcus, cryptosporidia (a rare bacteria), salmonella, and strongyloides (a tropical parasite) are some of the most common causes. These infections share the symptoms of severe diarrhea, malabsorption (which is the inability to absorb food), malnutrition, and bleeding of the stomach and intestines.

People in the late stages of HIV infection suffer from a wide range of illnesses in all parts of their bodies. While they are being attacked from the outside by infectious organisms, there are also conditions caused by HIV itself. The most common of these is abnormalities in all types of blood cells, causing unusual bleeding and anemia. Lymphoma (the cancerous growth of lymph tissue) also sometimes occurs in the lungs, intestines, and brain tissue. Kaposi's sarcoma, an unusual skin cancer once seen only in elderly men, is now also quite common in the final stage of HIV. It is the appearance of any of these opportunistic infections—but often the purplish spots on the skin of Kaposi's sarcoma victims—that leads a doctor to say an HIV-positive individual has AIDS. Weight loss and wasting away is another major problem in AIDS patients. Patients lose their appetite and ability to eat and suffer from malabsorption and malnutrition.

What is AIDS-related complex (ARC)?

Someone with ARC has a late-stage HIV infection but does not have the opportunistic infection or Kaposi's sarcoma indicative of AIDS. He or she may suffer generalized HIV symptoms like fatigue, fever, weight loss, diarrhea, and swollen lymph glands. Most people with ARC do later get an opportunistic infection, which signals the onset of AIDS. ARC is called a "pre-AIDS" condition and usually occurs in Stage 5.

Persistent generalized lymphadenopathy (PGL) is another "pre-AIDS" condition. It refers to lymph node swelling that is severe and extensive.

Isn't AIDS mostly a disease that gay men get?

The statistics on who has AIDS and how they get it vary by continent, country, city, and the particular study at hand. In Africa, more heterosexuals have AIDS than homosexuals. It is only in the U.S. and Europe that the bare majority of people with AIDS are homosexuals.

In the U.S. the statistics are changing, with new cases of HIV infection leveling off for homosexuals and bisexuals but increasing for IV drug users and the heterosexuals who are their partners. About 1.5 million Americans are HIV carriers, and 66,000 Americans already have AIDS. Sixty-three percent have been homosexuals, 19% IV drug users, 7% homosexual or bisexual men who used IV drugs, 4% heterosexuals, and 3% hemophiliacs or other recipients of contaminated blood in transfusions or blood products. The last 4% fall into no identifiable group. Of the cases in heterosexuals, 61% were known to have had sex with someone in a high-risk group, predominantly with IV drug users and to a lesser extent with homosexuals or bisexuals. The implications for women are important. In this group of those who had sex with a high-risk group member, three and a half times more women than men got HIV. This tends to support other evidence that it is easier for men to give HIV to women than vice versa.

HIV is not just a disease of adults or of any minority group, either. Children under thirteen who got it from their mothers in the womb were the fastest-growing group in the last year. Most of the mothers of these children contracted HIV through heterosexual sex with an IV drug user or were IV drug users themselves. Nearly 60% of all people in the U.S. with HIV are white, 25% black, 14% Hispanic, and less than 1% of other racial backgrounds. Since blacks make up only 11.6% of the U.S. population and Hispanics 6.5%, you can see that these groups have been struck very hard.

What is the AIDS test, and what does it test for?

An "AIDS test" does not test for AIDS, but rather for the human immunodeficiency virus, or HIV. The test, which is done by a lab using a blood sample, determines whether specific antibodies your body would produce in response to HIV infection are present in your blood. Being HIV-positive, therefore, means that a person *does* have these antibodies.

There are two tests used today, the ELISA and the Western Blot. The ELISA is done first, screening your blood for antibodies. If the first ELISA is positive, another ELISA is done on another sample of blood drawn at the same time. If this is again positive, the Western Blot, which is even more sensitive, is done. If the Western Blot test is positive, too, it is very likely (nearly one hundred percent) that the person being tested has HIV. If the first ELISA is negative, no further tests need to be done, because this test almost never fails to come up positive when HIV is present.

These tests are the good news: They are a quick, easy, and inexpensive way to determine whether or not you or your partner has HIV. The bad news is that there is a "window" of time when you test negative even if you've been infected. This is the period of time after infection but before the body has begun making antibodies (which the test detects) in significant enough numbers for the test to catch. Even immediately after being infected a person can pass on HIV to others. Yet it takes from two weeks to six months before the antibody test will show that infected person to have HIV, with most people testing positive within six weeks. This means that if you believe you've been exposed within the last six months, you should be tested twice: once two months after the exposure and again six months after the initial exposure. If you think you were exposed more than six months ago, you only need to be tested once.

Who should be tested for HIV?

If you think you've been exposed, you should be tested. This is the only way to tell whether or not you have HIV. You should consider having a test:

• if you had sex with multiple partners—especially if you've been the passive partner in anal intercourse, which carries the highest risk.
• if you've used intravenous drugs or had sex with someone who does.

- if you or any of your partners have had sex with a prostitute in the last ten years.
- if you've had a male lover within the last ten years who is bisexual or may be bisexual.
- if your lover or partner is HIV-positive or has HIV symptoms.
- if you or any of your partners have had a blood transfusion or used any kind of blood product before 1985.
- if you are the wife or partner of a hemophiliac.
- if you are pregnant or thinking about becoming pregnant and believe you may have been exposed in the past.

In short, being in a high-risk group or having sex with one or more people who are probably means you should be tested.

Even though you may be in a low-risk group, you may want to be tested for your own peace of mind. If you are beginning an intimate relationship with a new partner, a negative test for both of you (if the relationship is a monogamous one) may mean you can have sex more freely.

How and where can I get tested?

The test can be done by most medical testing labs throughout the U.S., but you do have to have blood drawn for it. Your own doctor can do this; if you don't have one, look in the phone book for the number of your local health department, usually found in the blue government services pages. The health department can either do the test or direct you to someone who does it.

It is very important that anyone who goes for testing also receives pre-test and post-test counseling. Your doctor or a health department counselor will tell you what the test does, how it works, and what the results mean. They can also help someone who has just discovered he or she is HIV-positive cope with the fact, providing important support and information.

What happens if I test positive for HIV?

If you've tested positive, you will no doubt be shocked and scared. Call your local AIDS hotline where knowledgeable volunteers can talk with you about your fears and direct you to the support services in your area. These organizations often have up-to-date information on treatment and may also be able to refer you to local doctors and hospitals with special expertise in HIV and AIDS.

If you or your partner do test positive, you need to find a doctor knowledgeable about HIV and AIDS, if you don't already have one. She will take a medical history to determine your general health and how you might have been infected. Your doctor will want to do a thorough physical exam, checking for enlarged lymph nodes and other irregularities of the skin and mouth. Blood tests, including a T-cell count comparing numbers of T_4 to T_8 cells, will help determine what stage of HIV infection you're in. The lower the number of T_4 cells, the more risk you have of developing AIDS and the more closely your doctor will want to watch you for signs of opportunistic infections.

If HIV and AIDS can't be cured, why should I get tested?

First, you should know that HIV is a very recent disease about which we know very little, compared to diseases like cancer that have been studied intensively for decades. Though we know how it is transmitted, who is getting it, and how to prevent it, the long-term effects of the disease—especially how many of those with HIV will get AIDS—are less clear. Today it is thought that many, though not all, of those who are HIV-positive will go on to develop AIDS, so a positive test does not automatically mean you will get AIDS. If you have HIV and don't know it, you could infect your partner or spouse and unborn children.

Finally, while there is no cure for HIV, there are treatments that retard its growth, but they depend on timely diagnosis to be effective. *Azidothymidine (AZT)* works by competing with HIV to get into the genetic code of the cells. Every cell whose genetic code AZT penetrates is another cell HIV can't take over to produce more copies of itself. In people in the later stages of HIV infection, AZT can actually increase the number of T_4 helper lymphocytes, protecting the body against further opportunistic infection and helping the person gain weight and strength. Though AZT can prolong the life of a person who has had AIDS for a year, it is thought that the drug is more effective if given earlier in the course of the disease. Researchers and drug companies are testing a myriad of new drugs to combat HIV. Right now, *early AZT treatment* gives the person with HIV the best chance to live longer and fend off the onset of AIDS.

Stress, poor health habits, and bad diet are known to affect immune functioning. The sooner the virus is detected, the easier it will be for your doctor to help you address these issues.

If I get tested, will others know the results, too?

HIV is a reportable disease, which means that doctors are required to report the results of the tests they do to local, state, or sometimes federal health authorities. However, there is also a widespread policy of permitting anonymous testing, in which a doctor submits a coded sample of blood and only the patient and doctor have access to the results. You might feel more comfortable going to a local HIV-testing site where your name won't be asked and your results will be recorded only by code.

Some states—Illinois, for example—now require couples applying for a marriage license to be tested. The results are reported only to the couple, not the state. Most insurance companies now require an HIV test for those applying for new life insurance policies over $100,000. Just about all disability policies—which pay you if you become unable to work—require an HIV test, too. No one—not a doctor, not a police officer—can require you to take an HIV test. The choice to get tested is yours alone. An informed decision—based on a knowledge of local testing and reporting policies—is crucial to protect your rights and safeguard your health. Laws and practices vary from state to state, but in some states, once your results are written in your medical records, an insurance company may read them and deny you insurance on the basis of HIV-positivity. To guarantee absolute confidentiality, go to a public health anonymous testing site; before you go, think carefully about whom you can trust to share the results with.

Because HIV is a reportable disease, the person who does the test—your doctor or laboratory health officer—is required to ask you for the names of your sexual contacts (or in the case of drug use, anyone you might put at risk). They will contact them to tell them that they might be infected but will not tell them your name. If you choose, you can notify them yourself first.

If my HIV test is positive, can I lose my job, health insurance, or apartment?

It is illegal for employers, insurance companies, and landlords to discriminate against you if they discover you are HIV-positive. If you are healthy and have no problems performing your work, no employer can dismiss you. No employer can make you take a test as a condition of employment—they must make the offer of a job first. You can always refuse the job if they then ask you to be tested. Companies are permitted to test employees if the intent is not to discriminate—for example, if they are doing a health survey or benefit analysis.

If you seek a life insurance policy in most areas

except California and Washington, D.C., the company offering the insurance can make you take an HIV test and decline to enroll you if the test is positive. Once enrolled in a plan, however, a company may not drop your coverage if they learn you are HIV-positive, or if they believe you are in a high-risk group. If you were not completely honest on the application about your medical history, however, they may be able to drop you on the grounds that your application was fraudulent. Many states prohibit insurance companies from denying health insurance to HIV-positive people as they prohibit the companies from refusing to carry people with preexisting conditions like a bad back or history of heart disease.

Are there any other advances against HIV on the horizon?

Though researchers are testing many other drugs in clinical trials, so far AZT is the most effective treatment. Attempts to develop a vaccine, which would prevent those inoculated with it from ever getting infected, are going on around the world, though to date these efforts have not been successful. The biological characteristics of HIV—the way it overpowers a cell by taking over its genetic code, its up-to-ten-year or longer latency period, and the fact that its genetic makeup changes so quickly as it mutates—make the development of a vaccine more difficult. There are also experimental difficulties because researchers can't ethically deny the drug they're developing to volunteers in a study where all are exposed but only some get the real vaccine in order to see if the vaccine prevents those inoculated from getting it.

Important advances have been made in treating the underlying infections in late-stage HIV and AIDS. A wide range of antibiotics have been successful in combating most opportunistic infections. Doctors have found that the sulfa drug *co-trimoxazole* and the drug *pentamidine* are effective against the once-deadly pneumocystis infections and their recurrence. Unusual varieties of tuberculosis are now being treated with newly developed antitubercular antibiotics. Though these powerful drugs can have serious side effects, they are allowing people with late-stage HIV to live longer and more comfortably.

How can I protect myself against HIV?

There are a few simple rules to lower your risk of getting HIV. Don't have sexual contact with anyone in a high-risk group. Know your partner; find out if he is or has been bisexual or an IV drug user. If you are worried, make sure he's healthy by asking him to see his doctor and have an HIV test. Limit the number of people you're sexually intimate with—a monogamous relationship with a healthy partner is the best way to avoid contracting HIV or any other STD. If you're an IV drug user, get into a treatment program and don't share needles or works.

We don't always feel comfortable asking those we have sex with questions about bisexuality, drug use, and their previous sexual history, and many men and women would think you were being alarmist if you asked them to have a test. Know that if you don't follow these guidelines, however, you are putting yourself at some risk. Still, there are ways of reducing that risk, and the best is always practicing safe sex with your partner. (See the safe sex chapter for complete information.) You may choose to have only "dry" sex, so called because it does not involve the exchange of body fluids. You may choose protected wet sex, which *tries* to prevent the exchange of bodily fluids with a barrier contraceptive like a condom for him and spermicidal foam or jelly for you. By now you have read how HIV is transmitted, and you know how you can get it. Knowing the risks should help you to make sound decisions about whom you have sex with and what you do with them.

CHAPTER EIGHT

Other Viral STDs

Though HIV is the viral STD that has attracted the most attention to date because of its grave consequences and the epidemic nature of its spread, **hepatitis B**, the **cytomegalovirus (CMV)**, and **Epstein-Barr virus (EBV)** are three other common viruses that can be sexually transmitted. In fact, there are more new cases each year of hepatitis B, which is transmitted like HIV in body fluids, than of HIV.

Hepatitis B

"Hepatitis" means inflammation of the liver, and **hepatitis B** is the name of the strain of virus known to cause this kind of hepatitis, which is also called serum hepatitis or long-incubation hepatitis.

People get hepatitis B through contact with the body fluids of someone infected with the disease. It can be transmitted through contaminated blood in dirty syringes and needles and hence is common among IV drug users. It is also sometimes transmitted by dental equipment, ear-piercing devices, and tattooing needles. Since all blood banks have screened for hepatitis B for many years, getting it from a blood transfusion is extremely rare.

Hepatitis B is present in the saliva, semen, vaginal secretions, feces, and blood of infected people. Therefore, it can be transmitted during vaginal and anal intercourse, deep kissing, and oral sex, though the latter two are not as risky for either passive or active partner as both kinds of intercourse.

Two to three months after getting hepatitis B general symptoms of severe fatigue, loss of appetite, nausea, vomiting, achiness, and headaches often occur. One or two weeks later the person becomes jaundiced—the skin and the whites of the eyes take on a yellowish hue because the inflamed liver is not getting rid of the pigment (colored substance) it makes, which it usually does when healthy.

Hepatitis B is diagnosed from lab tests that analyze liver function, with the specific diagnosis made on the basis of blood tests that look for the hepatitis B surface antigen—the virus particle—in the blood.

A person with hepatitis can feel very ill and completely fatigued, though the jaundice usually disappears after several weeks to a month. He or she will not be able to go about the tasks of daily life—going to work, taking care of children, etc.—for as long as four months after becoming ill. Most people recover, and though the disease is not usually life-threatening, it can be. About five percent of those infected will have long-term effects of a permanently scarred liver. A damaged liver can limit what you eat and drink, and those who have had hepatitis B liver damage usually can't drink alcohol without severe ill effects because the liver can't cleanse the body of it.

Not everyone develops the symptoms, though even an asymptomatic carrier will have the hepatitis B antigen in his or her blood. Such carriers, if they never have symptoms and aren't diagnosed, can unknowingly infect others. Some people—whether or not they have symptoms—will remain capable of infecting others with it for the rest of their lives, unlike the majority, who cease to be contagious once they have recovered. People who do carry it in an active, contagious state are called chronic carriers, and the condition is known as "chronic carrier state."

If you think you might have been exposed, or have symptoms, see your doctor. She will recommend complete bed rest for several months. There is no real treatment. During this time, don't have sex, because you can easily pass the disease to your partner (and ask him to get tested, too, since he may also have it). Because hepatitis is so easily spread, don't breast-feed, and avoid sex until your doctor gives you a clean bill of health.

Cytomegalovirus and Epstein-Barr Virus

The **cytomegalovirus (CMV)** and **Epstein-Barr virus (EBV)** are very similar in the symptoms they cause, how they're transmitted, and how they're treated.

EBV causes infectious mononucleosis, in which normal lymphocytes (white blood cells) undergo changes in their cell structure due to the virus. CMV affects lymphocytes, too, increasing their number and altering the ratio of T_4 to T_8 cells, somewhat like what happens in HIV infection.

Both viruses can be transmitted sexually, since the virus particles in the lymphocytes are found in saliva, semen, vaginal and cervical secretions, blood, and urine. Transmission can occur during anal and vaginal sex, oral sex, from blood transfusions, and through sharing contaminated needles and syringes. Other routes of transmission include shared eating utensils and other kinds of repeated casual contact, especially for those living in crowded conditions like boarding schools and barracks, where both diseases occur more often. Therefore EBV and CMV are not strictly STDs.

CMV and EBV are both diagnosed from blood tests that show higher than normal numbers of lymphocytes and evidence of "atypical" lymphocytes (with changes due to the virus) in blood cells viewed under a microscope. The diagnosis is confirmed by blood tests that reveal the presence of EBV or CMV antibodies the immune system manufactures in response to infection.

Several weeks after contracting either virus, an

infected person usually has symptoms of exhaustion, sore throat, swollen glands, or swollen lymph nodes all over the body—under the arms, in the groin, on either side of the throat, around the collarbone, under the chin. Since they are viruses, there is no real cure or treatment beyond getting plenty of bed rest. Most people recover within several weeks to several months with few problems. A small number may develop chronic mono or persistent CMV with fatigue or cold symptoms that won't go away or that return over time.

CMV during pregnancy or birth can be transmitted to the fetus, which occurs in about one percent of the births in the U.S. each year. Ten percent of these newborns have severe problems from the virus like blindness, mental retardation, and growth problems. Usually, transmission to the fetus occurs when the mother is having her first attack of CMV.

EBV or mononucleosis is very common. About ninety percent of the U.S. population has been exposed to mono at some time, though most don't get the symptoms. EBV and CMV do the most damage in people with malfunctioning or absent immune systems—people with lupus or HIV, or people taking certain medications (like prednisone for cancer treatment) that depress the immune system.

If you have or think you have EBV or CMV, see your doctor. She will advise you not to breast-feed or share eating utensils with others or to be intimate until the infection is over and symptoms have passed. If you've recently had CMV, you should not plan to become pregnant before your doctor has made sure that all infection is gone. If you are pregnant and get CMV, see your doctor immediately. She can tell you about the risks and will want to follow your pregnancy closely.

Though it is harder to avoid EBV, since it is so common in the general population, you can lower your risk of getting CMV and hepatitis B by practicing safe sex and being aware that both viruses are transmitted in the same ways as HIV, though neither virus is nearly as serious in its effects. This means that the risky sexual behaviors and risk groups are the same, too. Chapter 7, "AIDS and HIV," has complete information on what these risks are and how you can protect yourself.

PART V

Safe Sex and Birth Control

As we've seen in the preceding chapters, there are many kinds of sexually transmitted diseases and many ways to get them. This does not, however, mean you'll inevitably get one. By choosing a healthy partner and by practicing safe sex you have an excellent chance of avoiding *all* STDs. You've already taken one step forward and now know or can quickly learn what most common STDs look like and how they are transmitted. You've learned the importance of regular checkups for your sexual health and have learned some of the ways in which your body signals you that it's time to see a doctor. That's already more than most people know!

For STDs, even more than for other diseases, the old saying holds true—an ounce of prevention is worth a pound of cure. In the case of STDs, prevention focuses on *who* is your sex partner, *what* you do with him, and *how* you do it. Practicing safe sex means taking precautions in these three areas by knowing as much as you can about your partner's sexual history, by knowing what is safest (dry sex) and what is not (intercourse with no protection), and by using **condoms, spermicides, dental dams,** and other things to make the sex you do choose to have as safe and pleasurable as possible.

Birth control, because it shares a goal with safe sex—preventing one partner's bodily fluids from coming into contact with the other's—plays an important role in safe sex. Though not all methods of birth control are equally effective in protecting you against disease (the IUD actually increases your chance of getting one), which kind you choose to use is an important factor in your risk of getting many STDs.

CHAPTER NINE

Safe Sex

If you never come into contact with a disease, you can't get it. The first step in protecting yourself against STDs, then, is limiting the number of people you are intimate with sexually. If a person has sex with four people in a year, and they each had four other partners, that person is unknowingly exposed not only to the other four and their four partners, but to any disease of the partners of those four, and the partners they may have had . . . and the original person has been exposed to 256 people, though only having sex with four of them.

On the other hand, a monogamous person with a monogamous partner is exposed to her partner and his previous partners only—a risk that, for most diseases, declines very quickly over time if both people are in good health. Practicing safe sex at the start of the relationship makes that risk even less.

Monogamy is not for everyone, and many of us will choose to be intimate with more than one partner. The best way to avoid STDs is to practice safe sex whenever you are intimate—whether it is with the same partner for a number of years or with a new partner.

What is safe sex?

STDs are transmitted when one person's moist mucous membrane tissue comes into contact with that of another. It is the bodily secretions—semen, vaginal and cervical fluids, saliva, feces—that carry the infection to the vulnerable mucous membranes of the vulva, vagina, penis, anus, and, sometimes, the mouth. For sex to be safe there must be no mucous membrane contact between partners, and also no secretion contact. Secretion contact is, for example, when semen in a man's pubic hair brushes against a woman's vulva during a close embrace or when a man ejaculates into a woman's mouth during oral sex.

How do you have safe sex?

There are different kinds of safe sex that don't involve mucous membrane or secretion contact. Dry sex is the safest, with almost no risk of getting an STD or getting pregnant, because in this there is not even the potential for such contact (hence the term "dry"). When you have safe sex this way:

- you and your partner can kiss each other anywhere *except* for the mucous membrane areas—i.e., on the penis, vulva, nipples, or anus. Wet or French kissing is out, since it involves saliva exchange.
- you can rub against your partner clothed. Naked, you can rub your clitoris against your partner's arm or leg. He can rub his penis against your abdomen or thigh, but not near your vulva or anus.
- your partner can massage your breasts, nipples, vulva, and clitoris—any part of your body except your anus—with his hands and fingers. He should avoid touching his penis so that no sperm or ejaculative fluid (the clear fluid that escapes from the tip of the penis before ejaculation) or vaginal secretions are exchanged.
- you and your partner can each masturbate yourselves at the same time.

When you are having dry sex and are both naked it's a good idea for your partner to wear a condom from the start. Then, if he ejaculates, you won't have to worry that his semen might reach your vulva when you embrace. A condom is also a good idea if you want to touch or massage your partner's penis. Although STDs aren't contracted through tough, dry skin like that on your hands, if either of you does come into contact with the other's secretions, it's a good idea to wash immediately with soap and water. You should be especially careful if you have open sores or cuts on your hand or elsewhere on your body. Also, if you use a vibrator, make sure it is your own. If your partner has his own, make sure he hasn't used it with anyone else.

Keep the vibrator clean and disinfect it after use with mild soap and water. Remember not to use oil-based creams or lubricants when using a condom, since they will weaken it.

As you can see, dry sex lets you be very intimate but still very safe. "Petting"—dry sex when you're both clothed—is safer when you're with someone for the first time. With clothes on, there is no danger of secretion contact. Dry sex allows you and your partner to touch and have orgasms yet also feel confident that you're not putting yourselves at risk. Dry sex can be a good, satisfying alternative.

Is dry sex the only way to have safe sex?

Aside from no sex at all, dry sex is the safest. The alternative of wet sex, while never completely "safe," can be made safer if you are cautious. Wet sex is any kind of behavior in which penile and vaginal secretions or saliva are exchanged or that involves anal contact. Wet sex therefore includes vaginal intercourse, anal intercourse, oral sex, and deep or French kissing. Wet sex also includes any other way in which one partner comes into contact with the mouth, vagina, nipples, vulva, penis, or anus of the other partner, even without intercourse. Wet sex without protection can therefore be *risky*. For a monogamous couple in which both partners are healthy, wet sex is not risky. With a new partner, or if you and your partner aren't monogamous, however, unprotected wet sex puts you at significant risk for most STDs.

Wet sex is safe sex only when it is protected—that

is, when you use a condom properly and take other precautions. The **condom,** a thin sheath usually made of latex, fits snugly over the penis; it is a barrier method of contraception, but also a good preventative measure against STDs. This is because the condom provides a physical barrier between your partner's penis and your vulva, vagina and cervix, and anus. The condom prevents his semen from coming into contact with your vaginal and cervical secretions. Though not one hundred percent effective (they do sometimes break or leak), used with a spermicide they are the best protection you can have.

Before other contraceptives like the birth control pill and the intrauterine device (IUD) came into use in the 1960s, the condom was one of the only contraceptives available. When people stopped using condoms, however, the rates of STDs rose steadily throughout the population. Lately, given what people now know about AIDS, condoms have again become very popular. They are safe and easy to use and do help prevent most STDs. They are also the best way sexually active people can limit their chances of getting STDs without giving up intercourse.

Can oral sex be safe sex?

Though less risky than intercourse, oral sex is harder to make safe since by its nature it involves heavy contact between the mucous membranes of the mouth and those of the vulva or penis during which there is plenty of opportunity for disease organisms to pass directly from partner to partner in saliva, semen, and cervical and vaginal secretions. Unprotected oral sex is therefore *risky*.

There are two things you can do to make it less risky (you can't make it "safe") if you do choose to have oral sex. A man performing oral sex on a woman can use a **dental dam,** which is a very, very thin sheet of latex several inches square that is placed over the vulva. Like a condom on a penis, the dental dam forms a barrier so that his saliva won't reach the mucous membranes of her vulva and so her vaginal secretions won't reach the mucous membranes of his mouth. If your partner uses the dental dam, he must be careful that fluids don't escape around the edges or get on his hands or fingers, which may be close to his mouth as he holds the dam in place. He should wash his hands afterward, too.

A woman who wants to have oral sex with her partner can make it safer by having him wear a condom. She should make sure the condom stays in place and stop if her partner has reached orgasm. He should remove the condom and wash his penis and pubic area with soap and water before embracing his partner again intimately. She should wash her hands.

What's the correct way to use a condom?

First, you must use a condom every time you have sex for it to be effective. You may want to use a lubricant for intercourse with a condom. Some condoms come prelubricated, but if they don't, make sure you use a **water-based** lubricant, which you can find in any drugstore under the brand names *K-Y Jelly, H-R Jelly,* or *Today Personal Lubricant. Do not use oil-based lubricants like Vaseline or baby oil or most hand creams and moisturizing lotions; don't use saliva.* Oil-based lubricants will weaken the latex and make the condom more likely to break. Saliva can transmit STDs.

You or your partner should put the condom on his penis as soon as it becomes erect but before you have any intimate contact, even though you may just be caressing or cuddling each other. This usually isn't difficult since most men get erections from deep kissing or petting before you're both undressed. When you put on a condom before you have sex you prevent accidental contact between penis and vulva, especially of the fluid that escapes the penis during arousal but before ejaculation. You also won't be tempted to do without it as you become more aroused.

When you take the condom out of the package be careful not to tear it. Don't unroll it, but look for any holes, tears, or nicks. You can put a drop of lubricant on the head of the penis; this helps the condom slide on. Don't put lubricant on the shaft of the penis, though, since the dry shaft helps the condom stay on during intercourse. Some condoms have a reservoir—a little space at the tip to collect the semen—and these work best. For a condom without one, leave about one quarter to one half inch at the end. Gently grasping the reservoir or half inch of condom you've left (and pinching it so there's no air left inside), put the condom against the head of the penis and unroll it over the shaft. If your partner is uncircumcised, hold back the foreskin before you try to put the condom on. Make sure the condom is rolled down as far as it will go. When it is on, inspect it again for any tears or holes.

After orgasm your partner should withdraw from you immediately, holding the condom at its base to prevent it from falling off or leaking semen. You should both wash then, making sure vulva, penis, and pubic hair are thoroughly cleaned with soap and water. This is so any fluid that might have spilled from the condom doesn't come into contact with your vulva and so any of the secretions around your vulva don't reach his penis later.

Never use the same condom twice. If you have intercourse three times in an evening, you need three condoms.

What about condoms and anal sex?

Condoms were never designed to be used for anal intercourse, which puts more pressure on the condom because the anus is not as elastic as the vagina, nor does it have its own lubrication. However, anal sex with a condom is certainly safer than anal sex without a condom. Because this activity is the most risky in terms of HIV transmission and because secretion contact is much more likely from a broken condom, you should definitely avoid it, even with a condom. Anal sex is not safe sex.

Are some condoms better than others?

Condoms are made of either latex or lambskin (so-called natural or natural membrane condoms). Lambskin and other natural membrane condoms are thinner, and some people who use them claim that they allow a man to feel more pleasure. Yet these condoms, because they are thinner and made of a different material, may not be as effective against the transmission of AIDS and other STDs as synthetic latex condoms. Studies have shown that the AIDS virus cannot easily pass through a latex condom. To be sure, use synthetic latex condoms.

Some condoms come lubricated with *nonoxynol-9,* a spermicide used in foam contraceptives and with the diaphragm. Nonoxynol-9 has been shown to kill the AIDS virus on contact and is also effective against gonorrhea, trichomonas, and chlamydia. These condoms give you extra protection. If you can't get them, use a plain condom with a spermicidal foam contraceptive, which should be used before you start intercourse, not after.

Some condoms are not as well made as others, and some brands break more often. *Consumer Reports* (March 1989) rated the following latex condoms with nonoxynol-9 to be most reliable according to their tests: Excita Extra, Sheik Elite, Koromex with Nonoxynol-9, Ramses Extra with Spermicidal Lubricant, Lady Trojan, Trojan Plus 2, Lady Protex with Spermicidal Lubricant, Protex Contracept Plus with Spermicidal Lubricant, Trojan Ribbed, Wrinkle Zero-0 2000.

Even as you read this, condom research and technology is moving forward. Many companies are developing new materials and methods to make condoms more pleasurable and effective. The Japanese, for example, have recently been test-marketing a condom made of a new kind of ultra-thin but ultra-strong synthetic latex that is meant to withstand even the rigors of anal intercourse.

What can I do if a condom breaks?

If you are using condoms, you should also have on hand some spermicidal foam contraceptive. If the condom does break, you can quickly apply the foam, which will help kill the sperm and many common STD organisms. You should not douche, however, since this might only wash the sperm or disease organisms further up the vagina or through the cervix.

What if my partner objects to using condoms?

Though condoms are not the most elegant things in the world, they protect you from nearly all STDs. You and your partner can make them less a burden and more fun to use. Just as making love involves both of you, so does taking responsibility for birth control and safe sex. You can help him see safe sex as a shared experience by asking him to try using a condom with you, emphasizing that of course you'd rather be natural but that for now it's just not something you want to do.

Condoms don't have to be plain and ugly, either. They can be quite colorfully tinted, ribbed, contoured, and textured. You can try several of the highly rated brands to see what you both like. Tell him you'll help him put it on and let that be part of the experience. Make sure first—by practicing on your finger—that you know how. Tell him that lots of men find they can prolong sex and make it more enjoyable with a condom. Be creative! One woman presented a box of blue condoms to her new boyfriend all wrapped up with blue ribbon. "I knew blue was your favorite color," she told him. He didn't object. If all else fails, you can refuse to have intercourse without condoms.

What can I do to make practicing safe sex easier?

Half of the battle is being prepared and knowing what to do. Buy a package of condoms and keep some in your purse or pocket and some at home. If you are having an intimate dinner with a partner-to-be and think you may want to have sex with him, put a condom on your night table so that you won't forget to use it.

Safe sex is about making choices and being responsible for your sexual health. You are the one who chooses whom to be intimate with and exactly what you want to do with him. You should consider, in the beginning of a relationship, or if you think it might be short-term, having only dry sex and making sure your partner knows that you take safe sex seriously. You can be intimate without having intercourse or oral sex, and often taking longer to get to know each other isn't a bad idea. You may decide you don't really want to go any further. Or you might discover that learning how you can please yourself and your partner in other ways makes intercourse, when you do choose to have it, more exciting.

Don't make assumptions about a prospective partner. Just because he is neat and clean, went to a good college, and grew up in a nice middle-class family doesn't mean he can't get STDs and transmit them to you. AIDS is *not* only a disease of IV drug users and homosexual men. And as we have seen, other STDs like genital warts, chlamydia, and herpes are very common in young, otherwise healthy adults. You never know, and you can't tell. Take precautions.

What should I know about a prospective partner?

Before you become intimate with a man, it is your right to know the facts of his sexual history. You should know:

- if he is or was a sexually active homosexual or bisexual (even if it was a single encounter in previous years).
- if he or any of his past partners have ever used intravenous drugs.
- if he is a hemophiliac or received blood transfusions before 1985.
- if he is being treated or has recently been treated for any STD, especially conditions like genital warts or herpes.
- if he is HIV-positive.
- if he has ever been to prostitutes, here or in another country.

These are not the easiest questions to ask, and they may make both of you uncomfortable. But they are important questions—so important that they can save your life. If you don't think you can bring yourself to ask, think for a moment: Would you rather be uncomfortable or embarrassed for a few minutes or risk the possibility of disease? Honest communication is a vital part of safe sex and any good relationship. Remember, you have a right to safe sex.

What's the best way to talk to a partner about safe sex?

There are many ways to bring up the subject. Here are a few suggestions that may make it easier:

- First, decide on your personal ground rules, let a prospective partner know what they are, and stick to them. Think carefully about what is right for you and try to share your feelings honestly. You might decide to be intimate with someone only after you know all the answers to the questions listed above. You might choose to have only dry sex until you really know a partner well. Or you might decide you'll never be comfortable with a partner unless he (and you) has had an HIV test.
- Let prospective partners know right from the start that you are concerned about STDs and AIDS. You could begin to do this by talking generally about what you've read and heard, about friends you may know who've gotten an STD like herpes, and how *you* are concerned about your health and the health of those you choose to be intimate with.
- You are the best judge of the right time to talk about safe sex. It might be after several dates, when you

feel you know him well enough to talk about more personal things. It might be at lunch or over a drink after work. Try to choose a place and time that is private, when the focus is on intimate conversation rather than being intimate physically.

- Don't wait until you're in the bedroom, when expectations are already high and assumptions already made. If you find yourself in a situation you are uncomfortable with, stop!

- When you're talking to your partner about safe sex, be aware that he may get defensive. You can defuse this by underlining the seriousness of the consequences (which you will know after reading this book) and by reminding him that safe sex protects both of you. If he still does not get the idea, tell him that there is no choice involved; you find him attractive and sexy, but you don't have sex unless it is safe sex.

  Being asked if they are bisexual or homosexual is interpreted by many men as threatening their masculinity. You can reassure them ("I know you are attracted to women") while explaining that some people do experiment sexually and that it's something you need to know about.

- Hold your ground. If you suspect he's being less than honest, don't have sex!

Safe sex is *not* a life sentence; it *is* a way to approach being sexual with a new partner in a responsible, caring, and satisfying way. Safe sex offers choices that will help you enjoy a healthy sex life. If you've just met someone, dry sex is a good way to begin. When you know him better and are satisfied that he's been honest with you, you might want to be more intimate, having intercourse with a condom and spermicide. Eventually, if you're both monogamous and enough time has passed (and you've both been tested for HIV and had a checkup for other STDs) so that you know he's healthy, you can consider other alternatives besides a condom.

What should I do if a partner says he's used IV drugs, had sex with prostitutes, or been an active homosexual or bisexual in the past, but I still want to begin a relationship with him?

Because most HIV carriers are in those groups, you must ask yourself a very difficult question: Is it worth the risks to my health and life to become involved sexually with this man? That may seem melodramatic or hard to believe, but just remember that it is the wives and partners of male IV drug users, to take one example, who make up the largest group of women who have gotten HIV. They got it mostly through unprotected vaginal intercourse.

If you do choose to begin this relationship, don't have sexual contact with him until he's had an HIV test and a medical checkup. If he's tested negative in the past but engaged in high-risk behavior in the last six months, he should be retested. If his test is positive, you will both probably agree that your relationship should remain a celibate one.

Even if his test is negative, you still need to make some choices, because any sex—even by-the-book dry sex—puts you at risk. If he continues to do high-risk things, and you are having some kind of sexual contact, you both should have periodic HIV tests. Having sex without a condom in this situation is like playing Russian roulette—it's extremely risky, and it's very likely that you could get HIV.

Sex with a high-risk group member can never be safe. Even with a condom and spermicide, you are still tempting fate. Studies suggest that if you have sex with an HIV carrier and use a condom, you still may run as high as a one in five chance of infection. Again, remember that AIDS doesn't discriminate, and ask yourself if your health and your life are worth risking.

What do you tell your patients when they ask you about safe sex?

I tell them that it is irresponsible not to practice safe sex. Safe sex is not a matter of ego, power, or even feelings; it's an issue of health and life. No one has the right to object to your insisting on safe sex. And once you understand the principles behind safe sex and hold your ground on them, you'll find it gets easier. Once you're involved in a monogamous relationship, or when you've both been tested and had a checkup, you can begin to consider other alternatives.

Safe Sex Checklist

- Remember that safe sex is a matter of life and death.
- Consider limiting the number of partners you have. Safe sex with a healthy partner is best.
- Decide your rules first and stick to them.

- Buy some condoms and spermicide; carry them with you and keep some at home.
- Let a prospective partner know what you expect of him before you begin.
- Ask those important questions about his health and habits. Take the time to get to know a possible partner—that makes communication easier.
- When in doubt, find out—ask him to have a test or checkup first.
- Remember what is safe and what is not and don't be tempted when you've had a few drinks or if someone is very persuasive.

CHAPTER TEN

Birth Control

Which kind of birth control you use and how you use it can determine not only whether or not you get pregnant, but also whether or not you put yourself at risk for getting certain STDs. Barrier methods of birth control—the condom and the diaphragm—prevent pregnancy by creating a physical barrier that stops sperm in the man's semen from passing through the cervix into the uterus and tubes so that fertilization can't take place. Non-barrier methods like the birth control pill and intrauterine device (IUD) work by disrupting the body's normal processes. Though they prevent pregnancy better, they *don't* protect you from STDs. Choosing a barrier method of birth control and becoming comfortable and familiar with it are important steps in protecting yourself against both pregnancy and STDs.

Barrier Methods of Birth Control

Barrier methods prevent contact with your partner's bodily fluids, and this, you will recognize, is the idea behind safe sex. Barrier methods, used correctly, prevent STD organisms from gaining entry to the body and going on to cause disease just as they prevent semen from entering your body to make you pregnant. Barrier methods, unlike the pill and IUD, are the only kinds that give you this double protection, but they do vary in their effectiveness both in preventing pregnancies and in preventing STDs.

The **condom** completely covers your partner's penis and thus prevents any contact of his secretions with your vulva or vagina. Used properly and with spermicide, it can be the most effective of all birth control methods against the double problem of STDs and pregnancy.

Because both the **diaphragm** and **the cervical cap** allow the penis contact with vulva and vagina, it is easier to get an STD with these methods. Herpes and warts, for example, can both be transmitted when a diaphragm or cervical cap is used. So even though your cervix is covered by the diaphragm or cap, the protection given is not as complete as with the condom even against pregnancy. If you or your lover is not monogamous, it is safer to stick to condoms.

The diaphragm and cervical cap must also be used with **spermicide** or they are much less effective against both pregnancy and STDs. The spermicide nonoxynol-9, which is found in almost every brand, can not only kill sperm but also has some killing effect against gonorrhea, herpes, trichomonas, chlamydia, and, to a lesser extent, the AIDS virus.

Spermicides also have drawbacks whether they are used alone as foams, creams, or jellies or in suppositories and film or with a cervical cap or diaphragm. Spermicides can disturb the acidity of the vagina and make it easier for you to get certain kinds of vaginitis. If you already have vaginitis, they can make it worse. They also irritate the vagina, causing soreness, dryness, and, in the extreme, bleeding. They make it easier for you to get UTIs like cystitis and urethritis. Used alone, they offer far from one hundred percent protection against STDs and are much less effective than if used with a condom.

All barrier methods, because they involve putting a foreign body or substance in contact with the skin, can cause allergies and irritation. You can be allergic to the latex of condoms, diaphragms, and caps, which may make you itch when you use them. About one percent of latex product users are allergic. Between one and four percent of all spermicide users feel symptoms of irritation like burning, itching, swelling, or blistering. Changing brands can help, as can switching from foam to cream or vice versa. If the irritation is bad enough and persists, you might consider switching to another method of birth control. Talk to your doctor.

Some people say barrier methods are awkward, destroy the atmosphere of lovemaking, and interfere with romance and spontaneity. Some women find it hard to insert and remove a diaphragm, and some men say condoms reduce their pleasure. Spermicides often taste and smell bad to both men and women.

Yet for most people, the pros outweigh the cons. Barrier methods don't interfere with your body's functioning like the pill or IUD, but they provide good protection against STDs and pregnancy. They are extremely safe, and the problems they might cause in some women—vaginitis, urinary tract infections—are mostly minor and easily treated when they do occur.

The sponge, diaphragm, and cervical cap can cause one fairly rare but serious problem—toxic shock syndrome. Though TSS has mostly been found in users of certain kinds of tampons, there are a handful of cases that have occurred as a result of these three kinds of birth control. TSS is not an STD, and occurs when a common bacterium—staphylococcus aureus—multiplies rapidly within a foreign body like a diaphragm, manufacturing a toxic substance capable of causing a severe infection throughout the body. Symptoms include high fever, diarrhea, vomiting, muscle aches, foul-smelling vaginal discharge, and a rash like sunburn. Menstrual blood is a good place for the bacteria to breed, and this is why doctors recommend that you not use a diaphragm, sponge, or cervical cap during your period or if you have vaginal bleeding for any reason. You also minimize your risk when you take out the diaphragm, cap, or sponge when directed—don't forget and leave it in for long periods of time!

The Condom

The condom is also called a rubber, prophylactic, raincoat, hat, safe, French letter, or glove. It is a strong latex rubber sheath that looks like a balloon worn over the erect penis. See Chapter 9 for how to use a condom. Used correctly in combination with a spermicide, it is the best choice to accomplish the double goal of pregnancy avoidance and STD prevention. Some condoms come lubricated with nonoxynol-9, which can kill many disease organisms; they are therefore more effective than condoms without it. Don't use "natural" condoms (made of lambskin), because they are thinner and don't provide as good a barrier as latex. Very small germs like the HIV virus may be able to seep through lambskin condoms. The best condom to use, if you're going to use one, should have a reservoir tip (for the sperm) and be lubricated with spermicide. Many come already lubricated.

The pros are that condoms are relatively cheap, allow men to take responsibility for birth control, are small and easy to carry with you, don't require any "maintenance" or cleaning, and don't cause any side effects except in the case of allergy. They are believed to be effective in preventing transmission of chlamydia, warts, herpes, trichomonas, and gonorrhea, with some protection against HIV. Though condoms, like everything else, aren't completely protective against all STDs, they are the best protection you can have, especially if you use a diaphragm, too, when with a new or nonmonogamous partner.

The cons are that condoms have a twelve percent failure rate for pregnancy, which means that out of one hundred couples who use condoms for a year, twelve women will become pregnant. Some people say they interfere with spontaneity in sex; some men say condoms reduce the pleasure they feel.

Condoms can also break or come off inside you. If one breaks, immediately apply spermicidal foam or jelly. If a condom comes off inside you, pull it out immediately, grasping the open end to shut it. Insert spermicidal foam or jelly inside yourself and wash your hands.

As with any barrier method, you must use a condom each and every time you have sex. Remember, a condom is only effective when you use it correctly.

The Diaphragm

The diaphragm is a dome-shaped latex cup with a firm but flexible metal or spring rim around its edge. It completely covers the cervix, making a barrier between your partner's penis and your cervix. Since it does not cover the vaginal walls or vulva, it is less effective than the condom against most STDs, and especially against HIV. You can get genital lesion STDs (like herpes, warts, or trichomonas) when using a diaphragm, but the chance of getting cervicitis from STDs like gonorrhea and chlamydia is reduced—which lowers your risk of PID.

The diaphragm is best used with a partner you know well, preferably a monogamous one. When you correctly use the diaphragm and he uses a condom, you both get as close to one hundred percent protection as you can get against pregnancy and STDs.

You must have a diaphragm fitted to the size of your cervix by your doctor, who will help you choose one of three types: a flat spring, a coil spring, or an arcing spring. The difference is in the rim, and all are equally effective. The arcing spring is probably the easiest to insert; the flat spring has a rim that fits around the cervix more gently.

Size depends on the depth and width of the vagina and vaginal tone, and your doctor will fit you with the largest diaphragm that feels comfortable. He or she will show you how to insert it and help you practice putting it in and taking it out several times before you leave the office. Your doctor will also give you a diaphragm case, spermicidal jelly or cream, applicators, and an introducer to insert the diaphragm. You may need to be fitted with a new diaphragm from time to time, especially after having a baby.

The diaphragm is inserted into the vagina and pushed into place against the cervix before intercourse. Before inserting it you must put a heaping tablespoon of spermicidal jelly or cream in the dome (don't be stingy!) and spread it around inside it and over the rim for the diaphragm to be effective. Spermicide is effective for up to six hours, depending on the brand, but you must allow at least six hours after intercourse—not after putting it in—for it to do its work. This means you can insert your diaphragm up to six hours before having sex. Some women find that inserting it beforehand when they know or think they might have sex with a lover helps them to use it every time.

If your diaphragm has been in more than six hours and you want to have intercourse, you must either remove it and reapply spermicide or use an applicator to insert spermicide into your vagina. If your diaphragm is in and you've already had intercourse, you must use the applicator to reapply more spermicide if you want to have intercourse again. You can remove the diaphragm six hours after you last had intercourse. You must remove it within twenty-four hours; after that your risk of any kind of infection increases as time passes. It is best to remove it within twelve hours.

The diaphragm is usually easy to insert. After spreading the spermicide around the bowl of the dome, press the rims together so that the diaphragm folds. While standing with one foot up, or while squatting or lying down with legs apart, spread your labia apart and insert the folded diaphragm into your vagina. The rims should be toward the top of the vagina (so the spermicide doesn't come out). Guide it inward against the back wall of the vagina, curving it downward. When it reaches the end of the vagina you will feel it tuck into place over the cervix. Remember to push toward the small of your back as you're inserting it so that you follow the downward-curving path that is the natural shape of the vagina. If the diaphragm is inserted correctly, you shouldn't be able to feel it at all, except with your fingers.

If you have a coil-spring diaphragm, you can also use a plastic introducer. To use the introducer, put spermicide into the dome of the diaphragm and, with the cup up, squeeze opposite sides of the rim together. Slip one end into the notched end of the introducer and the other end over the notch that corresponds to the size of your diaphragm. With the cup up, push the introducer and diaphragm into the deepest part of your vagina and twist the introducer to release the diaphragm into place.

Always check to be sure the diaphragm is in place before having sex. The back rim should be tucked up behind your cervix and the front rim (nearest the vulva) beneath your pubic bone. You should be able to feel your cervix through the latex of the diaphragm as rubbery and firm. Remember that the spermicide goes on the inside of the diaphragm, the side facing the cervix. Check after intercourse, too, to make sure the diaphragm hasn't slipped out of place. If it has, don't try to adjust it but insert more spermicide immediately.

To remove your diaphragm, reach into the vagina and with your index finger pull the front rim down. Be careful not to tear it with a sharp fingernail. You can also remove it with the introducer. After each use wash it gently with plain soap and water, rinse it, and dry it. Store it away from heat. Don't powder it or get Vaseline or any other greasy material on it since that can wear away and weaken the latex.

The pros of the diaphragm are that it doesn't interfere with your body's natural functions, is reusable, causes few adverse side effects, and allows more spontaneity in sex than the condom, since it can be inserted hours before.

The cons are that the diaphragm has an eighteen percent failure rate for pregnancy, that it is not as good protection against STDs as the condom used with spermicide, and that it must be left in place for six hours after sex. Diaphragm users are also more prone to urinary infections and vaginal infections. Like the condom and other barrier methods, you have to use the diaphragm every time you have sex and use it correctly.

The Cervical Cap

The cervical cap, which has only recently been approved by the Food and Drug Administration, works much like a mini-diaphragm. It has about the same failure rate, too, around fifteen to twenty percent. It is a smaller latex cup that stays in place by suction. It is fitted and inserted much like the diaphragm, but since it is smaller and supposed to stick lightly to the cervix like a suction cup, inserting it can be more difficult. Also like the diaphragm, it must be used with spermicidal jelly or cream and must be left in place for at least six hours after intercourse. The care of the cap is the same as for the diaphragm: wash gently with soap and water; store away from heat.

Initially, it was thought that the advantage of the cap would be that it could be left in place for several days or even weeks. The caps available now, however, cannot be worn for such long periods of time and should be removed within twelve hours after intercourse.

Because the cap covers the cervix so closely, if you use it for a long time or very frequently for shorter periods, the cervix gets exposed to a pool of cervical secretions, spermicides, and any microorganisms that might have been present in the vagina and trapped against the cervix when the cap was inserted. Just as stagnant water lets mosquitos breed, the pool of liquid against the cervix may make infection and irritation more likely by giving it a place to grow. Because of this, if you are exposed to an STD or other infection or already have an infection and use the cap, you are probably more likely to develop a serious infection. Cap users may also experience more TSS than women who use other kinds of birth control.

Cautions for Diaphragm and Cervical Cap Users

• See your doctor if your cap or diaphragm becomes dislodged in the middle of your cycle, when getting pregnant is more likely.

• See your doctor at the first sign of painful intercourse, unusual vaginal odor and discharge, or bleeding or spotting between periods—these are all signs of injury and infection.

• Be aware of symptoms of bladder, vaginal, and urethral infections discussed in earlier chapters and see your doctor if you develop them. Some women who use these methods have an increased tendency toward infection.

• Be aware that some women who develop recurrent urinary tract infections or vaginal infections may need to switch to another method of birth control.

Foams, Creams, Gels, and Suppositories

Though the nonoxynol-9 octoxynol-9 contained in all the spermicides in foams, creams, gels, and suppositories is somewhat effective against some kinds of STDs and also kills sperm, these substances, used alone, have a high failure rate in preventing pregnancy: twenty-one percent for all women and up to thirty-two percent for younger women. Used alone, without a condom or other barrier contraceptive device, they are not much protection against STDs. Spermicides are much more effective against both STDs and pregnancy when used in combination with a condom, diaphragm, or cervical cap. This is because these substances don't kill all the sperm or disease organisms, and they lose their effectiveness over time.

When you do use one of these spermicides (and foam is thought to be better than either cream or jelly), timing is very important. Read the directions. Some can be inserted as long as six hours before intercourse, but most are effective only for an hour. If you have intercourse twice, even within the same hour, you need to reapply them.

Foams, gels, and creams require little preparation and can be ready to use in seconds. With foam, which comes in an aerosol can, be sure to shake it at least twenty times to mix it. Some brands require that two applicators full of foam be inserted into the vagina. Read the directions and follow them carefully.

If you use suppositories or VCF film (a glycerine sheet that releases spermicide when dissolved inside you), be sure to allow sufficient time—usually ten to fifteen minutes—for them to foam or melt. They must be placed deep inside you against the cervix. Your hands should be clean before touching the film. Douching is not necessary after using any of these products, and in fact you should not douche for at least six hours after intercourse when you use them. It is better that you don't douche at all. Instead of cleaning out the vagina, you may push a cervical infection farther up the genital tract. You will need an applicator for all foams, creams, and gels. Wash the applicator after each use with mild soap and water and store it in a clean, dry place.

The pros of foams, gels, creams, suppositories, and film are few: they are only somewhat effective against pregnancy, are relatively inexpensive, and do kill some kinds of STD organisms. The cons are that they are not highly effective in preventing either pregnancy or STDs when used alone. These methods can cause irritation and vaginal and urinary tract infections (from the chemicals in them). Many women find the odor and wetness of the products unpleasant and bothersome.

The Sponge

The sponge is a polyurethane disc that contains spermicide. One side of the sponge has an indentation to fit your cervix, while the other has a loop of nylon that is grasped to remove it. You can get it at most drugstores, sold under the brand name Today sponge.

To insert it, remove the wrapping and moisten it with about two tablespoons of water. Squeeze out the excess water and insert the sponge into your vagina against your cervix, with the loop side out and the dimple toward the cervix.

One advantage of the sponge is that after putting it in you can have intercourse as many times as you want within the next twenty-four hours and you don't have to add more spermicide. You must leave it in for at least six hours after intercourse. The longest you can leave it in is thirty hours. If you leave it in longer, it can irritate the vagina and cervix. This makes vaginal and cervical infection—and even toxic shock syndrome—more likely. Eventually, as hours go by, the sponge will dry up and crumble into pieces. You can remove them yourself with your fingers. Squatting helps. If you can't get it all out, go to the doctor.

The sponge, because it is a sponge, can also absorb natural vaginal lubrication, making you feel dry. Use K-Y Jelly or another water-based lubricant during intercourse to deal with this. Finally, sponges are not as effective in preventing pregnancy in women who have delivered babies, probably because the vagina gets longer and more stretched out after childbirth. The sponge does not fit these women well, so women who have had children should not use it. Overall, the sponge's failure rate in preventing pregnancy is about fifteen to twenty percent.

Non-Barrier Methods of Birth Control

Non-barrier methods of birth control include the **birth control pill** and the **intrauterine device (IUD)**. Both work by changing the way your body works to prevent conception. Neither the pill nor the IUD gives you any protection against any STD, and both, in fact, increase your chances of getting one.

The Birth Control Pill

The pill works by mimicking the effects of the female hormones estrogen and progesterone that your ovaries produce. The pituitary gland at the base of your brain releases hormones that cause the release of estrogen and progesterone, which prepare the uterus for fertilization. At the same time, the ovaries are ripening an egg that will descend into the fallopian tube. When you take the pill this process is interfered with, and the normal release of progesterone and estrogen does not occur, so no egg is released. As long as you take the pill your ovulatory cycle is suppressed by the small, steady doses of hormone taken every day in the pill.

The pill has been available for nearly thirty years, and long study and much clinical research have led to many reformulations. Today, the synthetic hormones used are in a much lower dosage, reducing to a large degree the number of complications women experience while taking it.

Common side effects of the pill include:

- short, light menstrual periods.
- fewer or no cramps during menstruation.
- mood changes like depression and decreased sex drive due to the effect of hormones on emotion.
- no PMS—many women on the pill don't have the irritability, breast tenderness, or fluid retention of premenstrual syndrome.
- spotting or bleeding between periods due to lower estrogen level; this may occur especially if you forget to take a pill or take it late; usually harmless, but your doctor will want to make sure it's not something more serious like infection or cervical problems.

Less common side effects include:

- nausea—uncommon; can be overcome by taking the pill at night vs. morning.
- weight changes (gain or loss); progesterone in the pill can cause bloating from water retention as in the

normal period; estrogen can cause changes in which body fat accumulates on body, increasing size of hips and breasts. Most weight change responds to good diet and exercise.

- improvement of acne; very rarely it worsens.
- chloasma, or darkening of skin pigment on the upper lip. This occurs in five percent of pill users but fades after stopping the pill.
- hair loss. This can occur while you are on the pill or even after you stop using it. Hair grows back slowly.
- altered blood test results for thyroid, blood sugar, cholesterol, liver, and vitamin and mineral levels.

Serious side effects of the pill are:

- liver problems like jaundice (yellowing of skin), which occurs in about 1 in 1,000 pill users. Benign liver tumors occur in 4 in 100,000 pill users, with symptoms of pain and swelling in upper right abdomen and weakness due to internal bleeding. Benign liver tumors increase a woman's risk of having a cancerous liver tumor.
- high blood pressure (hypertension). The pill causes the most cases of hypertension occurring as a result of taking medication.
- circulatory problems like blood clots. These occur more frequently in pill users since the pill alters body chemicals involved in clotting. Clots can form anywhere, usually in the veins of the leg or abdomen, and travel to the lung, blocking circulation. This is called an embolism and is very dangerous. Heart

attack, stroke, and blood clots are thought to occur more frequently in women who use the pill.

The risk for any of these serious complications increases with age and is worse for women who smoke. You should not use the pill if you smoke and are over thirty-five. If you are already on the pill, you should plan to stop taking it by age forty even if you don't smoke. Women who have ever had a blood clot or such circulation problems as irritation of deep varicose veins (phlebitis), stroke, or heart attack should not take the pill.

For women under thirty, especially those who don't smoke, the risk of having any of these serious side effects is small. Many find that because the pill is so effective in preventing pregnancy—about ninety-nine percent—the minor risks are outweighed by the benefits.

The Pill and STDs

The pill, because it does not prevent contact with your partner's secretions, will not protect you from STDs. While on the pill you should use a barrier-type contraceptive (the condom is best) if you and your partner are not monogamous.

The pill also causes changes in the surface cells of the cervix, making them more vulnerable to infection if exposed. This is called **ectropion,** which is a condition in which the tougher outer cells of the cervix are replaced by the more vulnerable cells of the inner cervix. Chlamydia, gonorrhea, herpes, and warts are more likely to be successful in invading these more delicate cells and infecting the cervix. But studies show that the pill does provide some protection against a disease that has already invaded the cervix going higher into the endometrium, tubes, and ovaries to cause PID. For some reason, PID infections are less common in pill users than in women who use no birth control.

The Pill and Cancer

Some doctors and researchers believe that women who take the pill have higher rates of breast cancer, but this has yet to be proven. The birth control pill, however, does protect against getting cancer of the ovary or uterus.

The rate of cervical cancer in pill users is about twice as high as that of women who use other kinds of contraception. Doctors believe, however, that it is not the pill that is causing the cancer, but rather that women who use the pill get more STDs like herpes and warts, which cause cervical atypia leading to cancer. Cervical cancer seems to occur more as a result of STDs than of anything else. Indeed, if women on the pill also use barrier contraceptives, they are no more likely to get cervical cancer than other women.

Who Can Use the Pill and How to Use It Safely

You should ask your doctor to prescribe the pill at the lowest possible hormone dosage to stop ovulation. The lower the dose, the fewer and less severe the side effects. To get the best protection against pregnancy and to prevent STDs, use a barrier contraceptive along with the pill unless you have no risk of getting an STD or are in a monogamous relationship. If you take the pill, it is my recommendation to see your doctor twice a year for a Pap test, blood pressure checks, and blood tests to determine how your liver is working.

You should *not* take the pill if:

• you have or have had high blood pressure, heart disease, stroke, circulatory problems, or blood clotting problems.
• you are over forty, or, if not already on the pill, are over thirty-five.
• you smoke; seriously consider quitting smoking and consult with your doctor.
• you have or have had liver problems or abnormal Pap tests, or if you've ever had cervical cancer.

The Intrauterine Device or IUD

The IUD is a small tab of metal or plastic that is inserted into the uterus by your doctor and left there, with a string hanging down through the opening in the cervix for removal. Millions of women used to use them because they were such an effective birth control method (only five to ten percent failure rate), could be left in for years once inserted, and didn't affect the spontaneity of lovemaking. In the 1970s, however, women began to notice the severe problems arising from pelvic infection the IUD caused, from infertility to massive infection throughout the body and even death. Lawsuits were filed, and many IUD makers took their products off the market. Today there is only one IUD available, though hundreds of thousands of women continue to wear older IUDs since discontinued by their manufacturers.

The IUD prevents conception (the meeting of egg and sperm) rather than ovulation like the pill. Inserted into the uterus, the IUD provokes a reaction from your body, which sends white blood cells (lymphocytes) to the site of intrusion by any foreign body—whether bacteria or disease organism or a metal or plastic IUD. Sperm trying to get through the uterus to the tubes are killed by these white blood cells as invaders, too. Even if a sperm made it through the hostile environment of the uterus to fertilize an egg in the fallopian tubes, that egg would be much less likely to implant itself on the uterine lining, which is constantly disrupted by the lymphocytes and other disease-fighting cells drawn by the IUD.

Because of the risks of pelvic infection from IUDs, nearly all doctors recommend that if you are wearing one, you get it removed. If you are choosing a new method of birth control, look somewhere else.

Among the IUDs women may still be wearing are the Dalkon shield (withdrawn in 1975), the Saf-T-Coil (withdrawn in 1983), and the Lippes Loop (withdrawn in 1985). If you have a Dalkon shield (it would have been inserted before 1975)—you should have it removed immediately, even if you've been perfectly healthy. Some doctors believe that the Saf-T-Coil and Lippes Loop can still be used if already inserted, but only under a doctor's supervision.

In 1986 two copper IUDs, the cu-7 (Copper-7) and Tatum T (Copper T) were discontinued by their manufacturers. As with the Lippes Loop and Saf-T-Coil, however, some doctors think you can continue to use one according to the guidelines and with your doctor's advice. Copper IUDs, though, rely on copper being released to be effective and stop being effective as they age. Since these copper IUDs only last three years, if you are wearing one inserted in 1986 (the last year they were made), you should have it removed anyway.

There is still one IUD available for new insertions—the Progestasert. It has a lower infection rate and causes fewer menstrual cramps (a common side effect of all IUDs). Because it releases progesterone, it must be replaced yearly.

Risks of IUDs

Once the IUD is in place, the normal environment of the uterine lining is disrupted. Even though the reaction caused by the IUD is infection-fighting, this chronic state can make it easier for you to get an infection if exposed.

Not all infections resulting from IUD use are caused by STDs. One possible source is the insertion itself, when bacteria from your vulva, vagina, rectal area, or even the examining room or instruments themselves can get into the uterus. Whether from insertion or an STD, most infections tend to occur in the first several months of IUD use. Such infections in the uterus spread easily to the fallopian tubes and ovaries, causing pus buildup, scarring, and infertility from blocked or damaged tubes.

If you get an STD while wearing an IUD, infection of the tubes and ovaries is very likely. Studies show that women who use IUD birth control have much more pelvic inflammatory disease than women who use other kinds of birth control. IUD users can get PID from chlamydia, mycoplasma, gonorrhea, and even herpes, which is rarely a cause of this disease in others. In women who don't use IUDs, such infections are more likely to stay in the cervix rather than migrating upwards.

Women who have such an infection will have all of the symptoms mentioned earlier in the section on acute PID. These symptoms include abdominal cramps, painful intercourse, bloody or foul-smelling vaginal discharge, and feeling sick with fever, chills, or achiness. Sometimes the IUD string, usually barely noticeable, will become shorter or longer or disappear altogether into the uterus.

Women who get pregnant while wearing an IUD are in a very serious and dangerous situation. Though getting pregnant with an IUD happens less than five percent of the time, it often leads to miscarriage. Since the IUD blocks the opening of the cervix, sometimes fetal remains aren't totally expelled from the uterus after miscarriage, causing massive infection very quickly. If you're wearing an IUD and miss a period or have abnormal spotting or bleeding between periods, see your doctor as quickly as you can. If you have unexplained fever, abdominal pain, or foul-smelling vaginal discharge, get to the doctor right away. This is an emergency that can't wait.

Half of all pregnancies that happen when a woman is wearing an IUD end in miscarriage. About one in three women who get pregnant and then have the IUD removed later have miscarriages. If a woman in this situation does get an infection, it is almost always fatal to the fetus and can be life-threatening to the mother.

Ectopic pregnancy—when the fertilized egg implants itself in the tube or elsewhere, instead of the uterus lining—is also found more often in women who use an IUD than in those who don't.

Sometimes the IUD can perforate, or put a hole in, the uterus lining while it is being inserted. Although this is rare, it can cause infection of the uterus and the whole abdomen and internal bleeding, with symptoms much like those of acute PID.

Other problems experienced by IUD users include more bleeding and more severe cramping during menstruation. If cramps are particularly severe or last for more than twenty-four hours, see your doctor—you may have an infection. Spotting or bleeding between periods also occurs. Sudden unexplained bleeding may happen when the IUD rubs against the uterine wall, bursting a blood vessel. If you notice spotting, see the doctor.

Any infection that occurs while a woman is wearing an IUD, whether she is pregnant or not, is a serious situation. Most often the IUD must be removed for the treatment of whatever organism is causing the infection to be effective. Any foreign body like the IUD is a breeding ground for infection.

Who Can Safely Use an IUD?

Women who can safely use an IUD:

- have one permanent partner who is also monogamous.
- have no risk of exposure to STDs.
- have been pregnant at least once.

- don't want to become pregnant again.
- have never had an STD, especially not a cervical infection.
- are over the age of thirty.

IUDs are risky unless you regularly see your doctor and can answer yes to all the conditions above. Using an IUD even in the best of circumstances is risky.

Non-methods of Birth Control

So-called "natural" methods of birth control like the rhythm method or testing cervical mucus provide no protection against STDs and very little against becoming pregnant. The rhythm method uses body temperature as a guide, with a rise of .3 to .5 degree indicating ovulation and thus a time for abstinence until the menstrual period. But things like fever, cold, or stress can affect body temperature, so pinpointing ovulation this way isn't a reliable guide. Testing cervical mucus involves examining your secretions every day. Mucus at ovulation is gelatinous, thick, and elastic and can be stretched between the fingers to several inches in length, providing an easy road for sperm to travel. This isn't always reliable either, however.

Ironically, both of these methods are used best to pinpoint ovulation when a couple is trying to *get* pregnant, not avoid a pregnancy. Neither gives you any protection against STDs, either.

Withdrawal, in which the man withdraws his penis from the vagina before ejaculation, is also unreliable since the few drops of fluid that escape the penis before orgasm contain sperm. Since there is no barrier between vagina and penis, this is very risky.

All of these methods put you at significant risk for getting STDs if exposed to them. None provide protection against unwanted pregnancy. Barrier methods are much better at accomplishing both goals.

Birth Control and Your Level of Protection against STDs

Very Safe: Condom and diaphragm used together with spermicide, used every time, used correctly.

Safe: Condom used with spermicide.

Moderately Risky: Diaphragm or cervical cap used with spermicide.

Risky: Diaphragm or cervical cap used without spermicide.

Sponge.

Spermicidal foam, jelly, cream, suppositories, or film used alone.

Extremely Risky: Birth control pill.

IUD.

No protection—rhythm/cervical mucus or withdrawal methods.

It is clear that the type of birth control you use can determine whether or not you will be at risk for getting certain STDs. By following the guidelines given above and consulting with your doctor you will be able to find a method that is safe and right for you.

Glossary of Terms

abdomen—area in the front of your torso from below your ribs to your pubic area. Contains vital organs such as the stomach, intestines, liver, spleen, and reproductive organs.

abscess—pus-filled cavity that occurs as a result of severe infection. A serious complication of PID.

acute PID—an infection of the pelvic organs when a woman feels very ill and has symptoms of fever, abdominal pain and tenderness, and vaginal discharge.

acute salpingitis—acute inflammation and infection of the fallopian tubes. Part of the PID syndrome.

AIDS (acquired immune deficiency syndrome)—a devastating disease that results in severe breakdown of the immune system and opportunistic infections.

anal intercourse—intercourse where the penis is inserted into the anus. Carries a high risk for HIV infection and other STDs with an infected partner.

anoscope—a long narrow tube with lenses at both ends. The doctor uses it to examine the rectal walls closely.

antibodies—infection-fighting proteins produced by the body's immune system in response to a particular infection.

anus—the small round opening in between the buttocks that leads to the rectum, through which feces pass.

ARC (AIDS-related complex)—a pre-AIDS condition with symptoms of swollen lymph glands, fatigue, fever, and weight loss.

ascending disease—a term used in this book to describe certain STDs that start in the cervix and move up to the pelvic organs.

asymptomatic—not showing any symptoms of a disease or infection.

Bartholin's duct infection—infection of one or both of the small Bartholin's glands located at the opening of the vagina. Not usually caused by STDs.

biopsy—tissue sample taken to diagnose disease.

birth control pill—an oral contraceptive taken daily. It works by preventing ovulation.

bladder—balloonlike organ that holds urine.

body fluids—semen, blood, cervical and vaginal secretions, breast milk, saliva, tears, and urine.

Caesarean section—surgical procedure by which a fetus is removed directly from the mother's uterus.

cervical atypia—microscopic changes in cervical cells.

cervical cap—contraceptive for women that works like a small diaphragm that stays in place over the cervix by suction.

cervical dysplasia—abnormal changes in the cervical cells that can precede cervical cancer.

cervicitis—inflammation of the cervix, often due to infection by STDs.

cervix—disclike connecting structure between the uterus and vagina.

chancroid—tropical STD that causes genital ulcers. Uncommon in the U.S.

chlamydia—bacterial STD that is now the most common STD among heterosexuals. It causes infection of the cervix and often spreads to the pelvic organs.

clitoris—knob of sensitive tissue at the top of the labia minora; becomes erect or blood-filled during sexual excitement.

colposcope—instrument used to diagnose disorders of the vulva, vagina, and cervix.

condom—thin sheath, usually latex, that fits over the penis to protect against STDs and prevent pregnancy.

condyloma lata—the genital lesion that occurs during the secondary stage of syphilis.

crabs—pubic lice; small insects that live in pubic hair.

cryosurgery—method for removing genital warts and treating cervical problems.

culture—small sample from an area thought to be infected that is "grown" in a lab. It indicates which, if any, infection you have.

cystitis—infection of the urinary bladder.

diaphragm—dome-shaped latex cup that covers the cervix; a barrier contraceptive, most effective when used with spermicide.

dry sex—sex that doesn't involve mucous membrane or secretion contact.

dyspareunia—painful sexual intercourse.

dysuria—burning feeling during urination.

ectopic pregnancy—when the fertilized egg attaches itself to tissue outside the uterus.

ectropion—condition in which the outer cervix is covered by cells that would normally be found in the inner cervix.

ejaculation—discharge of semen from a man's penis at the peak of sexual excitement.

ELISA—test that screens blood for antibodies. Used to diagnose AIDS.

endocervix—inner cervix.

endometrial biopsy—test in which a small sample of tissue is removed from the uterus, often to see if infection is present.

endometrium—uterine lining.

epithelium—type of tissue that lines the vagina, mucous membranes, and skin.

escherichia coli—bacteria in the feces that causes most cystitis.

estrogen—female hormone produced by the ovaries.

exocervix—outer cervix.

fallopian tubes—thin, delicate tubes connecting the ovaries and the uterus through which an egg passes to be fertilized.

fecal matter—solid waste.

feminine hygiene products—vaginal douches, deodorants, and sprays, mainly cosmetic, that can encourage infection by destroying the normal balance in the vagina.

fimbria—flared end of the fallopian tube. It draws out and delivers the egg from the ovary into the fallopian tube.

Fitz Hugh Curtis syndrome—a complication of gonorrhea and chlamydia that attacks the liver.

FTA—blood test for syphilis.

gardnerella—bacteria that causes at least half of all cases of vaginitis; can be caught by having intercourse with an infected man.

genital herpes—highly contagious and common STD that causes painful sores.

genitalia—external sex organs. Vulva in female. Penis in male.

genital warts—very contagious STD caused by the human papilloma virus.

gonorrhea—very common bacterial STD.

granuloma inguinale—rare STD found mostly in tropical and undeveloped countries.

heat cautery—method for removing genital warts.

hemophilia—a serious blood condition that requires frequent transfusions.

Herpes simplex 2—virus causing genital herpes.

HIV (human immunodeficiency virus)—virus that systematically invades and destroys the immune system that protects us from everyday infectious organisms. Also known as the AIDS virus.

HIV positive—having HIV antibodies in your blood signaling infection and the possibility of transmitting the virus to others.

infertility—condition of not being able to become pregnant or bear children. Often the result of STDs.

inguinal lymph nodes—small, round masses of tissue that drain fluids from the body.

in vitro fertilization—procedure in which an already-fertilized egg is surgically attached to the uterine lining.

IUD (intrauterine device)—birth control device placed in the uterus by a doctor; has a string that hangs down through the endocervix.

IV drug user—person who injects drugs with needles.

Kaposi's sarcoma—purplish spots on the skin that indicate AIDS infection.

kidneys—organs that lie in the small of your back on each side of the backbone. They remove poisons and other harmful waste from your body in the form of urine.

Klebsiella—bacteria found in the feces that can cause cystitis.

labia majora—large folds of skin-covered fatty tissue protecting the vagina and urethral openings.

labia minora—smaller folds of mucous membrane inside the labia majora.

lactobacilli—normal vaginal resident bacteria that help protect the vagina against infection.

laparoscopy—procedure in which a lighted tube is inserted in a numbed spot below the navel so that the pelvic organs can be closely examined.

laser surgery—sophisticated method for removing genital warts using a light beam.

lesion—bump, blister, ulcer, or sore.

LGV (lymphogranuloma venereum)—extremely rare STD mainly found in people returning from tropical, undeveloped countries.

liquid nitrogen—method for removing genital warts.

lubricant—preparation that lessens friction during sexual intercourse.

lymphocyte—a specialized white blood cell that fights off infection.

marsupialization—Bartholin's duct operation that makes future infections less likely.

masturbate—to excite by touching genitals or other sensitive areas.

menopause—body changes in a woman age forty to fifty when she stops ovulating and stops having menstrual periods.

menstruation—part of reproductive cycle when menstrual fluid, containing blood, is flushed out of the body.

molluscum contagiosum—the pox. A viral skin infection.

monogamous—having only one sex partner.

muco-purulent cervicitis—infection of the cervix often by STDs.

mucous membrane—thin pink tissue inside the mouth and nose, on nipples, urethra, anus, vulva in women, and tip of the penis in men.

mucus—normal vaginal secretion.

mycoplasma—bacterial STD that causes cervical and pelvic infection.

myometrium—muscular layer of the uterus.

NGU (nongonococcal urethritis)—any infection of the urethra in men not caused by gonorrhea.

opportunistic infection—common infectious organisms that take hold only because the immune system is weakened, as in AIDS.

oral herpes—canker sores, fever blisters, and cold sores.

oral sex—sex where contact is between mouth and penis or mouth and clitoris and vulva.

ovaries—major female reproductive organs that produce female sex hormones and eggs.

ovulation—release of the egg in women, generally fourteen days after the end of the last period.

Pap test—used on the cervix for the detection of cancer and other changes.

peritoneum—thin, strong lining of the abdomen.

PGL (persistent generalized lymphadenopathy)—severe and extensive lymph node swelling; a pre–AIDS condition.

pH—measure of how acid something is; used to diagnose vaginal discharges.

pharyngeal gonorrhea—gonorrhea in the throat.

physiologic leukorrhea—normal but persistent whitish vaginal discharge that is not a symptom of infection.

PID (pelvic inflammatory disease)—condition that is usually the end result of an infection like chlamydia or gonorrhea, which begins in the vagina or cervix and climbs up through the endometrium into the fallopian tubes.

post-sex vaginitis—vaginitis that appears a few hours after sex with itching and other symptoms. Often disappears on its own.

post-surgical PID—condition that appears when an already-present infection is stirred up and worsens to an acute PID after surgical procedure.

preseminal fluid—milky fluid that escapes from the tip of the penis before ejaculation.

proctitis—infections of the anus and rectum.

progesterone—female hormone produced by the ovaries.

proteus—bacteria found in feces that can cause cystitis.

pubic hair—hair covering the vulva.

pyelonephritis—infection of the kidneys.

rectum—the tube that leads from the anus to the rest of the intestinal system.

resistant infection—one that the usual antibiotics don't cure.

safe sex—protected sex when there is no mucous membrane contact or bodily fluid exchange between partners.

scabies—skin disease caused by the itch mite.

semen—liquid a man excretes at sexual climax that carries sperm.

sexually transmitted vaginitis—vaginitis generally transmitted by having intercourse with a man who carries the infection in the urethra of his penis.

Skene's glands—two tiny glands at the urethral opening that are noticeable only when infected.

sonogram—procedure that forms a picture of bodily organs on a TV screen by bouncing sound waves off them.

speculum—instrument used in pelvic exams to push back the vaginal walls so that the vagina and cervix can be examined.

spermicide—sperm-killing substance, usually nonoxynol-9, in cream, jelly, foam, suppository, and film contraceptives, used with barrier contraceptives or separately.

sponge—contraceptive in the form of a polyurethane disc that contains spermicide and fits over the cervix.

STD (sexually transmitted disease)—any disease given or caught via any sexual activity.

syphilis—bacterial STD. Easily curable if diagnosed early.

syphilis chancre—the syphilis ulcer. The first symptom of syphilis.

thrush—candida yeast infection of the throat associated with the immune system breakdown of AIDS.

traumatic lesion—scratch, scrape, or chafing on the genitals from everyday causes—may be red and itchy and may be caused by tight underwear or pantyhose.

treponema pallidum—bacterium that causes syphilis.

trichomonas—sexually transmitted protozoa that causes vaginal infection.

tubal or ectopic pregnancy—pregnancy in which the egg is fertilized and remains in the fallopian tube, which later ruptures. An emergency condition.

tubal surgery—surgical treatment to reverse the effects of PID scarring and infertility.

tubuloplasty—operation to reconstruct the tubes and restore fertility.

ureter—long tube that carries urine from the kidney to the bladder.

urethra—short, straight tube that carries urine out of the body through the urethral opening beneath the clitoris.

urethral opening—hole beneath clitoris between labia minora where urine comes out.

urethritis—infection of the urethra.

urinalysis—laboratory test performed on urine to detect disease.

urinary tract—four-part system including two kidneys, two ureters, a bladder, and the urethra, which creates, processes, and removes urine from the body.

urine culture—test that shows which bacteria are present in a sample of urine by creating ideal conditions for their growth.

uterus—major reproductive organ that nurtures the fetus during pregnancy.

UTI (urinary tract infection)—any infection of the urethra, bladder, or kidneys.

vagina—passageway, in women, between the inner reproductive organs and the outside.

vaginal discharge—any noticeable change in vaginal secretions.

vaginal intercourse—intercourse in which the penis is inserted into the vagina.

vaginal opening—opening to the vagina closely protected by the labia minora.

vaginitis—common inflammation or infection in women that occurs when the normal environment of the vulva and vagina is disturbed, usually by common bacteria.

VDRL—blood test for syphilis.

vulva—women's external genitals.

Western Blot—confirmatory test for AIDS.

wet sex—any kind of behavior in which bodily fluids are exchanged.

yeast—a type of fungus that is a common cause of vaginal infection.